Euthanasia and other Medical Decisions Concerning the End of Life

Information pertaining to this publication should be cited as being published in:

HEALTH policy

Volume 22/1 + 2 (1992)
Special Issue

Editors

Jan Blanpain (Editor-in-Chief), Leuven, Belgium
Mary E. Young (Regional Editor U.S.A. and Canada), Washington, DC, U.S.A.
Atsuaki Gunji (Regional Editor Japan and Asian Pacific), Tokyo, Japan
George Schieber (Reviews Editor), Baltimore, MD, U.S.A.

Editorial Board:

S. Altman, Waltham, MA, U.S.A.
G.F. Anderson, Baltimore, MD, U.S.A.
R.H. Brook, Santa Monica, CA, U.S.A.
J. Caldeira da Silva, Lisbon, Portugal
R. Chrzanowski, Aarau, Switzerland
K. Davis, New York, NY, U.S.A.
M. Defever, Leuven, Belgium
K. Emi, Tokyo, Japan
I. Forgács, Budapest, Hungary
J. Frenk, Cuernavaca, Mexico
D. Freund, Bloomington, IN, U.S.A.
S. Fujino, Tokyo, Japan
K. Groom, Reading, U.K.
K. Henke, Hannover, F.R.G.
B.S. Hetzel, Adelaide, Australia
W. Hsiao, Boston, MA, U.S.A.
D. Jolly, Paris, France
S. Kaihara, Tokyo, Japan
R. Klein, Bath, U.K.
A. Koizumi, Tokyo, Japan
P.R. Lee, San Fransisco, CA, U.S.A.
H.J.J. Leenen, Amsterdam, The Netherlands
A. Ludbrook, Aberdeen, U.K.
T. Marmor, New Haven, CT, U.S.A.
A. Preker, Washington, DC, U.S.A.
M. Prywes, Beersheva, Israel
U.E. Reinhardt, Princeton, NJ, U.S.A.
F.F.H. Rutten, Rotterdam, The Netherlands
R.B. Saltman, Atlanta, GA, U.S.A.
S. Sandier, Paris, France
F.W. Schwartz, Hannover, F.R.G.
K. Staehr Johansen, Copenhagen, Denmark
C. Wlodarczyk, Lodz, Poland

Euthanasia and other Medical Decisions Concerning the End of Life

An investigation performed upon request of the Commission of Inquiry into the Medical Practice concerning Euthanasia

P.J. van der Maas
J.J.M. van Delden
L. Pijnenborg

Department of Public Health and Social Medicine
Erasmus University Rotterdam
P.O. Box 1738
3000 DR Rotterdam
The Netherlands

in collaboration with the Central Bureau of Statistics, The Hague

Prof. P.J. van der Maas, M.D., Ph.D., is Head of the Department of Public Health and Social Medicine in the Faculty of Medicine and Health Sciences at the Erasmus University Rotterdam.

J.J.M. van Delden, M.D., is a Research Associate at the Centre for Bioethics and Health Law in the State University of Utrecht.

L. Pijnenborg, M.D., is a Research Associate at the Department of Public Health and Social Medicine in the Faculty of Medicine and Health Sciences at the Erasmus University Rotterdam.

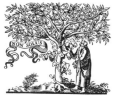

1992
ELSEVIER
AMSTERDAM • LONDON • NEW YORK • TOKYO

TABLE OF CONTENTS

Part II Physician interviews

Part III Death certificate study

x

Appendices:

Preface

This book describes the results of an investigation performed in The Netherlands during 1990 and 1991, on medical decisions concerning the end of life. From planning to reporting the investigation took only a little over a year. The impressive collaboration of a great number of physicians made it possible to gain, within this rather short period of time, good insight into the magnitude and the backgrounds of medical decisions concerning the end of life as they occur in The Netherlands. The medical profession appeared to be most willing to provide insight into one of the most difficult aspects of the practice of medicine.

We, the investigators, realised from the beginning that this investigation was not only to be a contribution to the discussion about legislation on euthanasia, but also had to contribute to the much broader public discussion about the important issue of medical decisions concerning the end of life. We received full support for this view by the "Commission of Inquiry into the Medical Practice concerning Euthanasia" chaired by Professor J. Remmelink. The intensive and pleasant collaboration we experienced on the part of this commission and its "Design of the investigation" subcommission was of great importance for the success of the investigation.

This book is an account not only of the Remmelink commission, but also of all physicians who collaborated with this investigation. We hope that the trust the medical profession put in our enterprise will be justified by this work.

The close collaboration with the Central Bureau of Statistics (CBS) deserves special mention. This collaboration yielded results that could not have been achieved by either of the research teams separately.

We carry the final responsibility for this report, although the investigation was designed, performed and reported in close consultation with the Remmelink commission and its subcommission. The conclusions the commission wishes to draw from this investigations are published in a separate commission report.

The work described in Chapters 11 (Sections 11.1 and 11.2), 12 and 13, in which design and results of the part-study performed by the CBS are described, was performed under the joint responsibility of the CBS and the Department of Public Health and Social Medicine of the Erasmus University of Rotterdam. A more detailed report of the CBS study is published by the CBS separately.

We started this investigation without preconceived opinions. We were convinced, however, that medical decisions concerning the end of life are an increasingly important aspect of the practice of medicine.

Although our task in this investigation did not go beyond establishing the facts as well as possible, we took the liberty of presenting in the final chapter some of the thoughts which we developed after a year of intensive involvement with the topic and many discussions with physicians.

The English edition contains the complete text of the Dutch version apart from a few minor adaptations.

P.J. van der Maas
J.J.M. van Delden
L. Pijnenborg

Acknowledgements

An investigation of the size described here can only be performed through joint efforts by a large number of people. We should like to express our sincere gratitude to those mentioned below. Some of these people have devoted much of their time to the entire, or to a large part of the investigation. A number will be co-authors of the publications that will appear in scientific journals. The names in each group are presented in alphabetical order.

Department of Public Health and Social Medicine of the Erasmus University Rotterdam
M.C.M. van den Akker, A.E. de Bruyn, J.M. Eimers, A.F.C. Gerritsen, A.G. Griffioen-Kisjes, J.D.F. Habbema, M.J.P. van Hooft, H.M. van Lamoen, C.W.N. Looman, J.P. Mackenbach, H.G.M. Rigter, D.R. Le Sage, Th.E. van der Starre-Bout, K.A.M. Wissink, and all other members of the Department of Public Health and Social Medicine who directly or indirectly made contributions.

The Dutch Central Bureau of Statistics
W. Begeer, J.T.P. Bonte, L.M. Friden-Kill, J.J. Glerum, A.Z. Israels, W.A.M. de Jong, J.W.P.F. Kardaun, P. Kooiman, M.F.P. van der Poel, S.J.M. de Ree, E. van der Schoor, E.J.M. van der Splinter, H.K. van Tuinen, P. de Wolf, and all other members of the Central Bureau of Statistics who contributed directly or indirectly.

The commission of Inquiry into the Medical Practice concerning Euthanasia, in particular the members of the subcommission on Study Design*
E. Borst-Eilers*, D. van Dijk, W.H.B. den Hartog Jager, A. Kors*. S.A. de Lange, J. van Londen, J.J.M. Michels, J. Remmelink, T.M. Schalken*, C.J.M. Schuyt*.

Advisors to the commission on Study Design
J.J.C. Pieters, C. Spreeuwenberg.

Interviewers

B.J.M. Aulbers, S.A. van Belle, A.E. Beukema, H. Blok, D.Ch.M. Gersons-Wolfensberger, C.A. de Geus, C.D. de Groot, L.J. Gunning-Schepers, C.P. van Heel, R.J. van der Hell, A.J.H. Hermans, W.G.J. Iemhoff, E. Iemhoff-van Kuilenburg, G.J. Kardolus, A. Klein, J. Knap, W.J.J. Ligtenberg, F.M.J.G. Martens, J.S. Meyboom, C. de Monchy, E.M. Nieuwenhuis-de Heer, S. Nijhoff, C.E.J. van der Post, J. van Rens, J.W. Schachtschabel, G.J. Schiethart, P.L. Schoonheim, F. Schreuder, A.J.B. Verkaaik, A.M. Vos-Kappelhoff.

And further

B.A. van Hout (Institute for Medical Technology Assessment, Erasmus University Rotterdam), A.B. Leussink (Dutch Health Council), P.G.H. Mulder (Institute for Epidemiology and Biostatistics, Erasmus University Rotterdam), W. Tijssen and J.P. Verouden (Office for Education, Training and Mobility, University of Amsterdam), F.C.B. van Wijmen (Department of Health Law, State University of Limburg).

Finally, special thanks are due to

all physicians who supplied data for this investigation: the physicians who collaborated with the test interviews, the hundreds of physicians who participated in the interviews and who then regularly completed questionnaires for several months, and the thousands of physicians who filled in the questionnaires circulated by the Central Bureau of Statistics.

This study was funded by the Dutch Ministry of Justice and the Ministry of Welfare, Health and Cultural affairs.

HOW TO READ THIS BOOK

Description and definition of concepts

In this investigation, the term *"Medical Decisions concerning the End of Life"* includes all decisions taken by physicians concerning actions performed with the purpose of hastening the end of life of the patient or decisions for which the physician has taken into account the probability that the end of life of the patient will be hastened. The actions concerned are: withdrawing or withholding a treatment (including tube feeding) and the administering, supplying or prescribing of drugs. Refusal of a request for euthanasia or assisted suicide and the decision not to resuscitate are also considered Medical Decisions concerning the End of Life for the purpose of this investigation.
This investigation does not consider:

– complications of medical interventions and medical errors in which hastening of the end of life was not at all envisaged;
– other medical decisions concerning the end of life, e.g. concerning the care of the patient, the possibility of letting the patient die at home, and all usual medical actions in which the (possible) hastening of the end of life is not an issue.

Considering the restricted meaning, as used in this investigation, of "Medical Decisions concerning the End of Life", the term has been capitalised throughout this text and has been abbreviated as MDELs.

The term "MDEL-action" is used in the description of the death certificate study and of the prospective study (Chapters 13 and 15). The definition of this concept is based on a combination of an action and an intention:

– the withholding or withdrawing of a treatment, either taking into account the probability that this decision will hasten the end of life of the patient, or with the explicit purpose of hastening the end of life;

– the intensifying of the treatment of pain and/or symptoms, taking into account the probability that this will hasten the end of life of the patient or in part with the purpose of hastening the end of life of the patient;
– the prescribing, supplying or administering of drugs with the explicit purpose of hastening the end of life.

He/she

Throughout the text, 'he' = 'she', 'his' = 'hers', etc.

Tables

Column percentages. All percentages reported in tables are column percentages, unless stated otherwise.

Rounding up or down. Percentages have almost always been rounded up or down to whole numbers. This implies that the sum of percentages referring to one particular total will not always be precisely 100. A number that became 0 due to rounding down is stated as "0". The absence of data for a certain class is indicated by "-".

Subtotals in italics. Several tables include subdivisions that are only applicable to one or part of all answer categories. If this subdivision is expressed as percent of the subtotal of these categories, the numbers and related text are printed in italics.

Missing values. When the number of missing values was relatively small and probably did not introduce bias, they were disregarded or distributed evenly over other categories. This refers especially to Chapters 5 to 10.

Weighting. Because the values were extrapolated in most cases to estimates for the entire Netherlands, the totals per row may not agree with the weighted average of the separate columns or rows. A percentage may also appear not to "fit" (e.g. a characteristic occurs in 3% of cases with n = 50). This is a consequence of the weighting procedure, which is discussed in Appendix E.

Appendices

The appendices are not numbered but carry letters. References to sections and tables in the appendices therefore carry a letter and a number (e.g.: "see Section E.3", "see Table C.2").

PART I

BACKGROUND AND DESIGN OF THIS INVESTIGATION

1. Reason and assignment

1.1 Introduction

Medical decisions concerning the end of life are being discussed increasingly frequently and intensively in many countries. In the United States discussion has focussed on non-treatment decisions. In The Netherlands euthanasia has been debated vigorously and publicly since the early 1970s, and this debate has attracted much international attention. Although euthanasia is a criminal act according to Dutch law, prosecutions are rare provided physicians abide by strict rules. Even so the physician often declares in cases of euthanasia that the patient died a natural death. The true number of deaths due to euthanasia in The Netherlands was therefore not known. Estimates differed a great deal and are often based on questionable factual material or on small numbers of observations. The publication of various important reports, books etc. certainly contributed to a better understanding of the problem, but the need for information about the actual occurrence of euthanasia in part prompted the investigation described in this report.

Impetus for the investigation also came from legal developments. Since 1973 several court decisions have concerned the question whether there can be a defence of justification regarding a charge under the sections of the penal code (293 and 294 respectively) that deal with euthanasia and assisted suicide. A legal consensus has emerged from these decisions that a physician can invoke a defence of necessity if he acted at the explicit request of the patient who was incurably and terminally ill and experienced prolonged and unacceptable suffering. A colleague is to be consulted to confirm the findings. The medical profession itself formulated 'rules of due care' with respect to euthanasia and assisted suicide. In the meantime, because of the opportunity provided by the courts, several proposals were made for reform to the law that forbids euthanasia and assisted suicide. From the mid 1980s on, one of the central questions in Dutch political debate was whether euthanasia should be legalized altogether, as proposed by some members of the Dutch parliament or should remain a criminal act in principle, but with clear rules about when not to prosecute.

The coalition government between Christian Democratic Party and the Labour Party that took office in 1989 decided to postpone the decision. In their agreement to form the coalition cabinet they stated that a Commission was to be formed that would report on the ''extent and nature of medical euthanasia practice'', ''based on the thought that there is no insight into the extent and nature'' of this practice. This was done by the appointment on January 17, 1990 of the ''Commission of Inquiry into the Medical Practice concerning Euthanasia'' by the Minister of Justice and the State Secretary of Welfare, Health and Culture.

The commission was charged with reporting on the state of affairs with respect to the practice of performing an act or omission by a physician to terminate life of a patient, with or without an explicit and serious request of the patient to this end. To perform its task, the commission would assign to a third party the task of performing an investigation directed towards obtaining insight into medical practice with respect to the problem of terminating life (acting or not acting) and into the factors that are of importance.

This report describes the investigation performed.

1.2 The history of this investigation

In a first discussion, at the end of February 1990, of the above mentioned commission chaired by Prof. Mr. J. Remmelink, with Prof. Dr. P.J. van der Maas, Head of the Department of Public Health and Social Medicine of the Erasmus University of Rotterdam, the following conditions posed by the investigator were accepted:

a. The investigator is responsible for reporting the results of the investigation. The report will be public. The commission is free to use the results for the production of its report;
b. There must be explicit collaboration of medical organisations, the chief inspectorate of the health supervisory service, the Ministerial Departments of Welfare, Health and Culture and of Justice, and possibly other institutions, e.g. the Central Bureau of Statistics (CBS);
c. No party may demand insight into data collected during the investigation in a form that might permit identification of any individual. The possibility of tracing individuals will exist only as long as is necessary for the investigation. The method for protecting individual data will be put in writing and submitted for approval to all parties concerned.

Several conditions determined the preparation of the assignment. The first was the instruction to the commission. It asked for quantitative information as well as for insight into the background of decisions and opinions of physicians. It was attempted to meet both these requests from the beginning. This could only be achieved by designing several part-studies within the context of one general investigation.

A second condition was the fact that the time available was limited. In principle, the investigation (including the report) would have to be completed before the summer of 1991. However it was clear to the commission and the investigators that the scientific quality of the project was not to be affected by the limitation on the time available.

The third fact was that it was necessary to collect new empirical data. It was certain that based on literature and registration data (for instance based on the cause of death statistics or on reports to the chief inspectorate of the health supervisory service) insufficient reliable data would be obtained. New data would have to be obtained from physicians who had taken relevant medical decisions concerning the end of life.

Based on considerations to be described below it was also decided to obtain the required information exclusively from physicians as respondents. It was accepted that only little justivce could be done to the views and experience of nurses and public. In spite of this, attention was paid whenever possible to nursing staff and the immediate circumstances of the patient.

1.3 The investigation: broad or narrow focus?

Much attention was paid to the question of whether the investigation should be aimed exclusively at euthanasia or also at other medical decisions concerning the end of life.

The following considerations led to the choice of the latter approach:

1. Although the word "euthanasia" occurs explicitly in the name of the commission, the commission's instructions suggest that other questions were also considered. These involved life-terminating acts other than acts upon explicit request of the patient and alleviation of pain and symptoms with shortening of life as side-effect. These two acts are not considered officially as "euthanasia" in The Netherlands.
2. There is a clear definition of euthanasia: "the purposeful acting to terminate life by someone other than the person concerned upon request of the latter" [1]. Nevertheless, there are several divergent interpretations of the concept of euthanasia in the medical profession [2]. A description of the topic of this investigation exclusively in terms of euthanasia could have led to estimates that might have been difficult to interpret.
3. The third reason for choosing a broad definition of the aims of this investigation was of a somewhat different nature and is related to recent medical developments. The number of therapeutic and life-prolonging procedures has been increasing steadily since World War II. As examples one might mention such widely differing items as medicaments (e.g., antibiotics), surgery (e.g., transplantations) and equipment (e.g., respirators). As physicians increasingly have such possibilities at their disposal, they will have to decide increasingly often whether to make use of these possibilities. A decision to withhold or withdraw a life-prolonging treatment can be as decisive in its consequences as administering drugs with the purpose of hastening the end of life. Moreover, the medical situation around the end of life will require the simultaneous consideration as to withdrawing or withholding treatment,

intensifying the alleviation of pain and/or symptoms, with shortening of life as side-effect and the administration of drugs with the purpose of hastening the end of life.

In the opinion of the investigators it was extremely important to be able to define the place of euthanasia within the entire scale of medical decisions which are taken when the end of life nears. The commission fully agreed with this view. Moreover, it was important to be able to decide between frequently occurring situations and exceptions. The literature contains a number of descriptions of individual cases. This complicates proper assessment of the relative importance of various kinds of decisions in terms of their frequency of occurrence.

1.4 Assignment

The commission formulated the assignment as follows:

− The institute (see below for explanation) is requested to investigate and report about the state of affairs with respect to the practice of acting or not acting by a physician with the purpose of hastening the end of life of a patient, whether the patient does, or does not, explicitly requests this. The report will be submitted at a date such that the commission can submit its report to the Minister of Justice and the State Secretary of Welfare, Health and Culture on May 1, 1991.
− The purpose of the investigation is to arrive at a reliable estimate of the number of cases of euthanasia in medical practice (acting to terminate life upon request) and of the number of cases in which life was purposefully terminated, by acts of omissions, without request.
− The investigation should reveal the characteristics of persons for whom euthanasia or termination of life without request was performed, of physicians who are involved and of the decisions that were taken.
− Moreover, the investigation should indicate the extent to which physicians were familiar with the rules of due care when decisions about euthanasia were taken and, if they were familiar with these rules he extent to which, and how, these rules were applied in practice.
− Finally, the conditions have to be studied under which physicians would be prepared to report truthfully thateuthanasia or purposeful termination of life without the patient's request was carried out.

The institute mentioned in above assignment was the Department of Public Health and Social Medicine of the Erasmus University in Rotterdam. In addition, the commission has requested the Central Bureau of Statistics (CBS) to perform a part-study on a sample of death certificates. It was agreed that in addition to this joint report the CBS would also publish independently about their study of death certificates [3].

Two further points merit attention. This investigation describes the views and the actions of physicians. It was intentional that no opinion was expressed about the acceptability of acts or of omissions. Moreover, there is a difference between the formulation of the task of the commission installed and the assignment for the investigation described in this report. The task of the commission installed involved the investigation of actions performed or omitted by a physician that lead to the end of life of the patient. In the assignment for this investigation the task was the study of the acts performed and omitted with the purpose of hastening the end of life. The subject of the investigation was thus limited because complications due to diagnostic or therapeutic interventions and so-called medical errors which can unintentionally lead to the end of the patient's life are excluded from the investigation. Thus, investigators and commission feel that they have followed the intention of Minister and State Secretary.

2. Design of the investigation

2.1 From assignment to design

The formulation of the assignment offered many possibilities for the actual design of the investigation. The development of the definite design of the investigation is described in this section.

The investigation had to meet six important conditions:

1. Quantitatively correct estimates had to be presented of the incidence of euthanasia and other important decisions.
2. Characteristics of the patients and physicians involved and circumstances under which decisions were taken had to be described.
3. Information about knowledge and views of physicians had to be collected.
4. The investigation had to provide insight into euthanasia and other important medical decisions concerning the end of life, in particular the purposeful termination of life by acts or omissions without request of the patient.
5. The amount of knowledge of physicians concerning the rules of due care with respect to euthanasia and its translation into practice had to be investigated.
6. Conditions had to be explored under which physicians would be prepared to report euthanasia truthfully.

Moreover, the timing for production of the report had to be such that the commission could submit the report to Government on May 1, 1991. This last condition could not be met; the report was submitted four months later. The two most important reasons for this delay were that the specialists' address file did not contain enough information to allow appropriate respondents to be selected in advance (see further Appendix C) and that so much valuable material was obtained due to the good collaboration on the part of the medical profession that more detailed but also more time-consuming reporting was justified. Fourteen months elapsed from the beginning of the investigation to completion of the report.

Clear definition and application of concepts

Medical Decisions concerning the End of Life (MDELs) take on a near infinite number of aspects. They are made in a situation in which the condition of the patient, the medical and technical possibilities, the psychic and social backgrounds of the patient and those of the physician all are important. However, some characteristics which are always of particular significance consistently emerge in these, always unique, circumstances . This became apparent during the discussions of both medical and social import. Examples are the capability of the patient to assess his situation and to take a decision adequately and whether the patient has, or has not, made an explicit request. The investigation therefore attempted to describe as well as possible the great diversity of MDELs, with particular attention to the essential medical and legal aspects.

To guarantee the clearest possible definition and application of concepts it was desirable to interview respondents (physicians) personally. Face-to-face contact between physician and well-trained interviewer was therefore part of the design of the investigation. Written questionnaires that present advantages such as guaranteed anonymity, efficient collection of large amounts of information and the total absence of a possible influence of the interviewer on the respondent, were also used extensively in this investigation.

Estimates

The degree of reliability of estimates is not only important for answering questions about numbers of cases of euthanasia and other important decisions. It is at least as important to clarify what are common situations and what are exceptions.

Recording the numbers of relevant decisions is not the only essential for making reliable quantitative estimates. Similar reliability is required for estimating the total number of deaths connected with the above mentioned relevant decisions. For instance, physicians can be asked if they ever have performed euthanasia and, if so, how often this has happened in the past two years. However, in order to present an estimate for the whole of The Netherlands, it is essential to know on how great a fraction of the total number of deaths the statements of the physicians in the sample are based. This latter information cannot always be obtained.

It follows that it is of interest to take a clearly defined sample from the total number of deaths occurring in The Netherlands within a given period of time and to find whether euthanasia or other important MDELs played a major role. A minimum of several thousands of deaths need to be studied to obtain a sufficiently large number of important MDELs.

It is clear that, considering the limited amount of time available for this investigation, it was not possible to both hold detailed and profound interviews with physicians and take a sample of several thousands of deaths. This investigation was therefore split into several parts (part-studies).

Backgrounds of decisions

It was considered extremely important that the many weighty aspects of MDELs should be considered. Estimates of the number of decisions actually taken should be seen in relation to the question of why a physician, in a particular case, prefers one type of action to another. Insight into this question can bestbe obtained by interviewing in detail, verbally, practicing physicians about the backgrounds of their decisions. Moreover, the question is of interest as to the extent to which the views of the interviewees about MDELs influence their practice of medicine in general.

Broad questions

In the previous chapter it was stated that the commission finally decided to consider the broader group of MDELs rather than limit itself to the investigation of euthanasia (Chapter 1). This does not imply, however, that equal attention could or should be given to all types of decisions. It was definite that euthanasia (terminating life upon the patient's request) and purposefully terminating life, by act or omission, without the patient's request, had to be described as well as possible. Situations somewhat further removed from these types of decisions could be described in broader outline.

2.2 Selection of the group of respondents

At least five groups of respondents had to be considered: physicians, nurses, pharmacists, institutions (hospitals, nursing homes, etc.) and the public. The final decision was to approach physicians only. The considerations leading to this choice are outlined below.

Physicians

It was obvious from the start that physicians had to be approached: the assignment of the commission was to report on the situation with respect to actions or omissions by physicians. Obviously, physicians would be the most direct informants. Moreover, it was obvious that physicians had to be interviewed who carried the complete responsibility for their decisions. Therefore physicians still in training were not included in the sample.

Nurses

There is no doubt that nurses play an important role in MDELs, particularly in hospitals or nursing homes. Through their daily and intensive contacts with the patient they will receive important signals earlier and often can evaluate the total situation better.

Nevertheless, there were several reasons for not drawing a sample of nurses. First of all, there was the assignment to the commission in which the physician and not the nurse was mentioned. The investigation was therefore focussed on the actions taken by the physician who is responsible in final analysis for the medical treatment and the decisions involved.

Also, it is technically very difficult, if not impossible, to draw a random sample of nurses as there is no file in which data on all nurses can be found. Moreover, many nurses will not be confronted directly with MDELs or involved in making decisions.

There were also other practical reasons which it was imperative to take into account in making this decision. The amount of time and effort involved would have been greater than was available within the short period available for this investigation. However, nurses' representatives were consulted when questionnaires were designed and the questionnaires to be used for verbal interviews with physicians incorporated as far as possible questions about the role of the nurse in the various decisions taken.

Pharmacists

While, in several instances, pharmacists are aware of the preparation or carrying out of euthanasia, they often are not. Therefore it did not appear necessary to interview pharmacists, either for reliable quantification or to obtain an insight into the background for this type of decisions, although they might be able to provide interesting additional information in a number of cases.

Institutions

Many institutions (e.g. hospitals, nursing homes) have a policy with respect to euthanasia. Could one assume that formal policy and actual practice do not differ greatly, studying institutional policies would then yield an impression of the actual practice. However, the correctness of the above assumption cannot be demonstrated in advance.

Also, there became available during the first phase of this investigation the results of another study that concerned institutional policies with respect to euthanasia [2]. This supported the decision of not aiming the investigation at institutions.

The public

There was intensive discussion about whether information obtained from an enquiry among the public would be necessary in addition to the information obtained from physicians. It was eventually decided not to draw a sample from the public. The most important consideration was that it would have been a very difficult way to obtain reliable information. It is often only a small number of those directly involved who know exactly what has happened in the case of a death. Also, it is very difficult to relate this type of information to an estimate of the total number of deaths about which the particular informant has relevant information. The impossibility of guaranteeing a reasonably consistent handling of concepts based on information so obtained or of arriving at sufficiently reliable quantitative estimates pleads against this approach.

Moreover, the questions to be asked could have a profound effect on the life of those involved who come from the immediate surroundings of the deceased. Recall of the situation around the end of life would be an emotional load to which the relatives should not be exposed except in the event of extreme necessity. There was no such necessity.

This, however, does not mean that obtaining information from this group would not have been important. On the contrary, it has often been demonstrated that communication between physicians and patients is far from smooth. Explanations regarding the illness and, e.g., the pattern of behaviour to be followed by the patient often appears not to be clear to the patient. It is thus obvious that, in the case of MDELs, particularly high demands are made of the ability of the physician to communicate. It cannot be excluded that relatives feel that consultations had not been particularly satisfactory while the physician was of the opinion that everything had been satisfactorily arranged with good understanding on the part of everyone. This aspect, however, is not part of the question central to this investigation.

2.3 Three part-studies

A three-part design was finally settled upon.

1. A sample was drawn from a population of physicians, to be defined further. These physicians were approached and asked to collaborate with an interview (retrospective study, physician interviews).
2. A sample was drawn from all deaths in The Netherlands within several months and the treating physician was asked to supply a limited amount of data about this death. The resulting death certificate study was performed by the Dutch Bureau of Statistics.
3. The physcians who had been interviewed (study 1) were also asked to record a small amount of data for any death that would occur in the subsequent six months and for which they would be the treating physician. This constituted the prospective study.

It was to be expected that certain situations in which decisions were taken would not occur sufficiently frequently to be reflected in the three part-studies described above. For such cases, which fall into special categories because of patient characteristics (e.g. being unable to take a decision) or illness characteristics (e.g. AIDS), complementary information was obtained from a number of experts from the areas concerned. Areas concerned include neonatology, other pediatric specialties, psychiatry and AIDS.

Retrospective study: physician interviews

A sample was drawn from general practitioners, nursing home physicians and specialists practicing in The Netherlands, the latter to the extent to which they are involved regularly in problems related to MDELs. The specialties involved were: internal medicine, pulmonology, cardiology, neurology and surgery. Nearly 90% of all clinical deaths fall under these specialties. As nearly one half of all deaths occur in hospitals and non-hospital deaths are almost 100% covered by general practitioners and nursing home physicians, this approach to selection of physicians covered about 95% of all death cases. Information about the 5% thus excluded was obtained from the death certificate study and from discussions with the experts mentioned above.

More than 400 physicians made up the sample. They were interviewed in detail (average duration about 2½ hours). Items discussed included:

- characteristics of the physician, such as specialty, type of practice, philosophy of life;
- requests for euthanasia and assisted suicide the physician had been concerned with in the period just elapsed;
- considerations about acceding or not to this kind of request in relation to its medical, social and legal context;
- other relevant situations in which decisions as to performing life-terminating acts or omissions were taken (to withdraw or withhold life prolonging treatment);
- factual examples of situations in which the physician had to take a decision himself;
- wishes concerning the nature and contents of regulations concerning euthanasia and other acts terminating life;
- considerations, in relevant cases, as to reporting or not reporting in the death certificate that a non-natural death was involved.

The interviews had to contribute to quantification. This implied extremely careful estimation not only of the incidence of important decision points, but also of the total number of death cases the physician had been concerned with in the period selected. The design of this investigation and its results are described in Chapters 4 to 10.

The death certificate sample

To strengthen the quantitative basis of the investigation a sample was drawn from individual deaths, in addition to sampling physicians. The best basis for such a sample is the death certificate file of the Central Bureau of Statistics (CBS). This file includes the data for all deaths of residents of The Netherlands. A so-called stratified sample was drawn that included about 8500 deaths. This number was chosen such that reliable estimates could be made of the number of cases of euthanasia and other relevant decisions, assuming that the sample had been drawn carefully and that the response of the physicians involved was satisfactory. The treating physician was identified for each death certificate included in the sample. This physician received a short questionnaire from the CBS, the so-called standard questionnaire. After completion this questionnaire could be returned completely anonymously.

The design of this study and its results are discussed in Chapters 11 to 13.

The prospective study

The physicians participating in the retrospective study were asked during the interview if they would complete a standard questionnaire for each died patient for which they, as the treating physician, had been responsible in the next six months. This standard questionnaire was identical to that used in the death certificate study.

The purpose of the prospective study was to support the quantitative estimates of the various MDELs obtained from interviews and death certificate samples as retrospective studies should always consider the possibility of some memory distortion.

Chapters 14 and 15 contain discussions of the design and results of this prospective study.

Complementary interviews

It is clear that several groups will be missed, even with the interviews of the size described and the death certificate study. The average number of deaths in certain specialties is so low that they do not appear in sufficient frequency in the sample of deaths. Similar problems would arise in a random sample of physicians working in these specialties. Based on these considerations, discussions took place with several physicians working in the missing specialties. These physicians could be assumed to know their fields of work and could provide information not only about themselves but also about the field in general.

Quantitative estimates could not be derived from these discussions but they did provide relevant descriptive information.

2.4 Instruments used for measurements

The information compiled in this investigation was obtained largely by means of two instruments: a questionnaire for theinterviews and a so-called standard questionnaire used for both the death certificate and the prospective study. The questionnaire for the interviews was very detailed – it covered more than 120 pages – and therefore is not presented in full in this book. The structure of this questionnaire is discussed in Chapter 4, while the formulation of the crucial questions is given in the text in conjunction with the relevant tables. The standard questionnaire is presented in Appendix A.

By sheer accident it may have happened that one particular physician was approached more than once. Thus it could have happened that someone received an invitation for an interview from the Erasmus University and also was asked by the CBS to provide written information about a particular death case. In such situations there was no question of the particular physician doing unnecessary extra work. Both parts of the investigation contributed, along different channels, to the information that was required. It was not possible to track down the respondent by combining information provided through different channels.

2.5 Privacy and data protection

Utmost care was given to the protection of privacy of the deceased, the participating physicians and the relatives and to ensuring the security of the data obtained in the course of the investigation. In the case of the sample of death cases, the CBS made arrangements such that absolute anonymity of both physician and deceased patient could be guaranteed. Procedures concerning mailing and assessment of data within the CBS made it impossible to track down the identity of either physician or deceased patient.

All data from interviews and the prospective study were made anonymous upon their receipt. Here too the data could not be traced back to particular respondents or patients except by a procedure that was known only to the investigators. The procedure for data safeguard was presented in writing to the respondent and was signed by the interviewer. The commitment was made that nobody could obtain any data, except in anonymous form and only for the purpose of scientific study. The information obtained has not been used for any purpose other than answering the questions asked in this study. In this way the guarantee could be given that the study would present no legal consequences for the participants.

2.6 Cooperation of the medical profession

Good cooperation by the medical profession was a prime requirement for success of this investigation. Credibility of the results would be seriously damaged should the response rate be low. Several steps were taken to encourage acceptance by the medical profession.

1. Protection of the privacy of physician and next of kin and the guarantees for the protection of data as discussed in the previous section were a prime condition for broad acceptance.
2. The Chief Inspector of the Health Supervisory Service and the Chairman of the Royal Dutch Medical Association (KNMG) wrote a letter addressed to all physicians in The Netherlands informing them of this investigation. They asked the physicians to cooperate if invited to do so (Appendix B).
3. Publicity in the general media was purposely kept to a minimum before and during the investigation. On the other hand, the study was carefully presented in the Dutch medical journals prior to its start. These communications were apparently read widely. Reprints of the paper in the Dutch Journal of Medicine (NTvG) [4] were sent to respondents in advance of the interviews.
4. A brief recommendation by the Chief Inspector of the Health Supervisory Service and the Chairman of the Royal Dutch Medical Association was enclosed with all invitations for interviews and questionnaires mailed by the CBS.
5. Almost all interviews were conducted by physicians.
6. The physicians who were to receive a standard questionnaire were written to by the Medical Officer of the CBS. This official was assisted by physicians posted at the CBS.

Moreover, the Royal Dutch Medical Association put the condition that it would support this investigation only if an instruction procedure concerning reporting and police actions in cases of euthanasia was produced.

The commitment by the Minister of Justice that such a guideline would be produced probably contributed to the willingness of the medical profession to cooperate.

2.7 Trial investigation

It is obvious that an extensive and detailed pilot study should precede a investigation of the purpose and aim as described. After some hesitation the investigators have agreed to forego a complete pilot study, in view of the very tight schedule.

A number of trial interviews were held during the development of the interview questionnaire which led to adjustments of the questionnaire. Also based on experiences in the interviews with general practitioners the questionnaire was slightly altered for the interviews with nursing home physicians and specialists. The standard questionnaire had to meet very high requirements because it had to be completely understood by the respondent without the presence of an interviewer, also it could only be tested to a limited extent by the investigators. Therefore it was decided that, during the first few weeks of the death certificate study, the responses would be inspected immediately upon their receipt, so that the questionnaire could be adjusted if necessary. Adjustments indeed turned out to be desirable.

3. Concepts and definitions

3.1 Introduction

The concepts that play an important role in this investigation are the subject of this chapter. Explanations are offered for the description and classification of different kinds of decisions. Several issues had to be taken into account for the choice and the description of concepts:

1. The entire spectrum of medical decisions concerning the end of life had to be included into the concepts and definitions to be used in this investigation. Defining what is and is not euthanasia was not sufficient.
2. This investigation is a description of actions by physicians and not a judgement regarding the acceptability of these actions. Therefore concepts, definitions and terms were chosen that are descriptive without any suggestion of value judgements, whether implicit or explicit. It was nevertheless not possible to completely exclude morally charged terms in a investigation of this nature.
3. Because the subject of this investigation was the physicians' actions and the physicians themselves were the respondents in this investigation, it was important to select concepts and classifications that fitted into physicians' patterns of thought and decision taking. This approach was not without important consequences. Differences, that are relevant for physicians may be of little relevance to legal experts and vice versa.
4. The results of the investigation had to be such that they could contribute to the discussions required for drafting legislation. This meant that findings should be classifiable into categories appropriate for this purpose.

Nevertheless, whatever classification is selected, there will always remain problems of delineation, of borderline cases or situations. These borderline situations are discussed in Chapter 17, in which estimates derived from the three different studies are compared.

3.2 Medical Decisions concerning the End of Life

Description of concepts

The term ''Medical Decisions concerning the End of Life (MDELs)'' as used in this investigation covers all decisions by physicians concerning courses of action aimed at hastening the end of life of the patient or courses of action for which the physician takes into account the probability that the end of life of the patient is hastened. The (courses of) action(s) concerned are: withdrawing or withholding treatment (including tube feeding) and administering, supplying or prescribing of drugs. Refusal of a request for euthanasia or assisted suicide and decisions not to resuscitate are also included in this investigation of medical decisions concerning the end of life.

This investigation is not concerned with:

– complications of medical interventions or "errors" that carry no intent to hasten the end of life of the patient at all;
– other MDELs, e.g. concerning the care of the patient, the possibility of allowing the patient to die at home, and all usual medical interventions where (possible) hastening of the end of life is not under consideration.

In view of the limited definition of the concept "Medical Decisions concerning the End of Life (MDELs)" as given in this section, this term will be spelt with capital initials and will be expressed throughout this book as the abbreviation (in capital letters) MDELs.

3.3 Classification of MDELs

The decisions we intended to research were classified on the basis of four important questions:

1. What does the physician do?
2. What is the physician's intention in doing this?
3. Did the patient request this intervention?
4. Was the patient able (or not) to decide upon this intervention?

What does the physician do?

Within this classification the physician can perform three interventions: administer "drugs" that (possibly) hasten the end of life, withhold or withdraw a (possibly) life prolonging treatment. Combinations of these interventions will occur frequently. If the aim is to shorten life by administering drugs it is obvious that life prolonging treatments will be withdrawn or withheld. Terminating a life prolonging treatment can sometimes lead to administering possibly life shortening drugs.

Persons other than the physician can be of importance. Self-administration by the patient of a drug prescribed or provided by the physician is a case of assisted suicide. Persons other than the patient or physician can also administer such a substance, e.g. nurses or close relatives. Euthanasia in which exclusively persons other than the physician perform the actual intervention is only considered in this investigation if the substance used was prescribed or provided for that purpose by the physician.

The physican's intention

This concept is one of the most difficult ones that had to be applied for this investigation. It will only be discussed here in general terms.

It can be assumed that termination of life can never be the most important aim in the interaction between physician and patient. If a physician deliberately performs actions that shorten the patient's life it can be argued that, in final analysis, termination of the patient's suffering is intended and that under certain circumstances, also according to the physician's judgement, this suffering cannot be terminated in any way other than by termination of life.

With respect to the physician's intention three categories were recognised for this investigation:

- (acting with) the explicit purpose of hastening the end of life;
- (acting) partly with the purpose of hastening the end of life;
- (acting while) taking into account the probability that the end of life will be hastened.

The first and third categories can be distinguished clearly. If a physician administers a drug, withdraws a treatment or withholds one with the explicit purpose of hastening the end of life, then the intended outcome of that action is the end of the life of the patient. This will not be the case if the action is performed while taking into account the probability that the end of life of the patient is hastened. The possible subsequent death may not have been intended.

This distinction of two major categories still does not solve the difficulty that many physicians cannot always indicate what their intention actually had been in a certain case. Sometimes an intervention is performed to achieve one particular effect (e.g., pain relief) but the side-effect (e.g., death) is not unwelcome. Strictly speaking, this situation should be categorised as intentional intervention. In order to be considered unintentional, this side-effect should in fact not have been desired. This strict interpretation could not be adhered to when the questionnaire was constructed because there were occasions when, in the opinion of the physician neither description did justice to his intention. We therefore allowed for the third category (acting) partly with the purpose of hastening the end of life. This description relates to a situation in which death of the patient was not foremost in the physician's mind but neither was death unwelcome. This type of intention was included specifically in the questionnaire for the alleviation of pain and/or symptoms.

The patient's wish

The patient's request is crucial for the discussion of MDELs. The (explicit) request of the patient even forms part of the definition of euthanasia [1,5,6] as used in current language of public health law. The term euthanasia is appropriate only once the patient requests an intervention to terminate life, perhaps making this request byof means of a written advance directive. The patient's wish is also important when a medical intervention is not carried out. As permission is needed for all medical interventions, refusal by the patient implies that these may not be carried out.

However, the patient's request must meet certain requirements, certainly if it concerns a request for euthanasia. The draft law on euthanasia from 1987 mentions 'a request made and adhered to voluntarily and after careful consideration' (art.6 para.2 sub c). The board of the Royal Dutch Medical Association included in their position on euthanasia the term "explicit" in the definition of euthanasia. Moreover the board mentioned the permanent desire to die as one of the rules of due care [5]. In agreement with the foregoing the concept "explicit request" is used as dividing line.

Other forms of expressing a wish can be distinguished in addition to the explicit request, e.g., on hearing an ominous diagnosis, a patient can ask his physician if he would be prepared to terminate life if, in due course, suffering would become unbearable. The patient absolutely does not intend that any action should be undertaken at that moment and in a number of cases there will never be a request for direct intervention. This situation was expressed in the interview questionnaire as a "request to perform euthanasia or assist with suicide in due course".

However, even if a request to terminate life within a foreseeable period of time is involved, one can distinguish between a request made spontaneously and an explicit and repeated request. The concept "request to terminate life in the foreseeable future" is used in the interview questionnaire, with further differentiation allowed for by means of additional questions.

The judgement of the patient

In addition to the definition of the manner of acting and of the request, the concept "(un)able to take a decision" plays an important role in our classification. This is a dificult concept because there is as yet little agreement about the criteria for the inability to take a decision [7]. A well-known legal definition is that someone is unable to take a decision if he is not able to reasonably appreciate his interests (preliminary draft law on surrogate decision-making), but we consider this definition less suitable for our purposes. Based on the available (mainly Anglo-saxon) literature the concept of 'being able to take a decision' has been defined as 'able to appreciate the nature of (assess) the situation so as to reach a decision adequately'. It should beemphasised that this description gives no criterion as to the outcome of the decision but does so only for the process of arriving at the decision. To do justice to the many aspects involved the questionnaire also allows for a situation in which someone was partially able to assess the situation and on this basis adequately take a decision.

3.4 Euthanasia and assisted suicide

In the previous section MDELs were classified on the basis of two pairs of concepts concerning physician and patient. This did not involve a strict definition of euthanasia. Nevertheless, this investigation will, in due course, have to provide a link to what will eventually be defined as euthanasia. The concepts of euthanasia and assisted suicide have therefore been used in several places in this investigation.

When the term euthanasia was used, it was used according to its accepted definition in The Netherlands. Euthanasia thus has been defined as the purposeful acting to terminate life by a person other than the person concerned upon request of the latter [1]. Assisted suicide, also in line with this State committee, is defined as the purposeful assisting of the person concerned to terminate life upon request of the latter. By using these definitions, the most important point of difference has become the person that performs the act of terminating life. In the first instance it is another person who performs the act, in the second one it is the patient himself. This distinction has been followed in this investigation. This implies that the role of the physician differs to the extent that in case of euthanasia the physician administers the drug or has it administered and in the case of assisted suicide he prescribes or supplies the drug.

3.5 Extent of shortening of life

The concepts 'terminal phase' or 'concrete expectancy of death' played an important role in the discussion of euthanasia. There was great resistance against the use of this concept as criterion for the admissibility of euthanasia. This, however, does not imply that such a concept would not be of importance in the taking of a decision. This is an important consideration, particularly for physicians.

To avoid use of these two controversial concepts, the question was formulated in this investigation so as to ask by how long, in the opinion of the physician, the life of the patient was in fact shortened by the action taken. This question was answered in most instances, both during the interviews and in the standard questionnaire, albeit with some hesitation.

There is no doubt that any estimate of the extent of shortening of life can only be very general. In practice, therefore, physicians are very reluctant to give an estimate of the length of time the patient is still expected to live. The estimates of the extent of shortening life as reported in this investigation certainly have no absolute value and should be interpreted with the greatest of caution. If, however, in a large number of cases the physicians indicated that life was shortened by a maximum of hours or days, the cautious assumption can be made that the patient was dying. If, in another type of decision, physicians indicated that life was shortened by weeks or months, one can assume that seriously ill patients were involved who were not yet dying. This investigation shows that the extent of life shortening estimated by the physicians differs markedly, depending on the type of MDELs. This indicates that more is involved than a relatively casual estimate.

Concerning withholding or withdrawing treatment it can be commented that the decision was to not prolong life by a certain period of time rather than to shorten life by the same period of time. The correct terminology depends on whether or not the results of usual medical treatment are considered part of human life expectancy.

3.6 Medically futile

A comment should be made in this discussion of the concepts used about the concept medically futile therapy. This concept plays an important role in the non-treatment discussion, with or without a request of the patient. Jurisprudence has appeared meanwhile in which this concept has been used. There is nevertheless no uniform definition [7,8]. The concept of 'futile' depends too much on what is considered to 'have a point', i.e. to make sense. This concept was therefore not used in the questionnaires because its interpretation is too variable.

3.7 'Do not resuscitate' decisions

In some situations there is an explicit agreement that the patient will not be resuscitated if a (functional) cardiac and/or respiratory arrest occurs. This anticipating decision is called a DNR (do not resuscitate) or NTBR (not to be resuscitated) decision. Such decisions play an important role in clinical practice. In this investigation they are also considered as an MDEL.

PART II

PHYSICIAN INTERVIEWS

4. Design and carrying out of the physician interview study

4.1 Introduction

This chapter describes the procedures followed for interviewing physicians. Items to be discussed are: selection of the respondents and drawing of samples, the construction of the questionnaire, response and quality control.

4.2 Selection of respondents

Study population

A sufficiently large number of MDELs have to be recorded in order to be able to present a reliable picture of the situation. It is obvious that a sample should be drawn from among persons acting regularly as the responsible physician in cases of death.

Several criteria had to be taken into account to decide what kind of physician was to be approached:

— there should be available a file of the types of physicians to be selected from which a sample could be drawn;
— the most important types of situations in which decisions have to be taken should be amenable to investigation.
— important groups of diseases should be sufficiently represented in the sample drawn;
— the total selection of specialties should cover most death occurring in The Netherlands;
— the number of relevant situations in which decisions have to be made should be sufficiently large in the sample.

Based on these criteria and on data about the distribution of deaths over the various types of physicians it was decided to include the following types of physicians in the sample to be drawn:

— general practitioners;
— nursing home physicians;
— cardiologists;
— surgeons;
— internists;
— pulmonologists;
— neurologists.

The latter five specialties cover some 30% of all clinical specialists, but the physicians in these groups are the responsible physician for 89% of all deaths occurring in hospitals. One should appreciate that oncologists (cancer specialists) are included among the internists. By sampling general practitioners, nursing home physicians and the above mentioned five specialties information is obtained that, in principle, covers 95% of all deaths in The Netherlands (see Appendix C).

Important situations in which decisions had to be taken will, however, have occurred in the remaining 5% of deaths, e.g. in neonatology and psychiatry. Physicians working in these areas are confronted with too few deaths in each year to be approached via a random sample, but they do have very specific experiences related to MDELs. A distinct approach was followed for several of these groups and is discussed in Chapter 16.

Anesthetists should be discussed separately. They are often involved in the treatment of pain and symptoms and it also happens that the anesthetist is asked to administer drugs in cases of euthanasia. In most instances, however, the anesthetist is not the treating physician. Respondents were asked in the interviews to describe also those cases in which they had been the most important treating physician but had delegated the performance of euthanasia to someone else, regardless of whether this person was an anesthetist or a nurse.

Other types of specialists are not included in the sample. The number of deaths in each of the specialties is small while the type of situation in which a decision had to be taken does not deviate to any great extent from situations occurring in the specialties selected. Adding a small number of respondents from other specialties probably would not contribute important information.

By limiting the sample of clinical specialties to the five already mentioned there are sufficient respondents for each specialty to allow several general statements to be made that apply for each of these specialties.

Sample size

The planned sample size included 410 respondents. These 410 respondents were distributed as follows.

The general practitioner is directly involved in almost half the deaths. More than 40% of the deaths in The Netherlands take place outside the clinic or nursing home. Also, this classification assigns deaths in which no physician was involved (e.g. a traffic accident) to the general practitioner. In spite of the fact that general practitioners cover more than 40% of cases, less than 40% of the sample was assigned to general practitioners. First of all, the work situation of general practitioners is fairly homogenous. Moreover, relatively more is known about MDELs in general practice in The Netherlands than in the other practice situations. It was therefore decided to include 150 general practitioners in the sample.

The sample size for nursing home physicians was set at 50. Individually, they are involved in the largest number of deaths annually, so that a smaller sample size is sufficient for an overview of a large number of deaths. Moreover, nursing home patients are a relatively homogenous group with respect to morbidity and age distribution. Also, it was to be expected that the number of MDELs would be relatively high in nursing homes.

The remaining 210 respondents were specialists. When determining the sample sizes of the five specialties mentioned earlier a distinction was made between internal medicine and the other four specialties. Internists are the largest group of specialists and are in attendance for more than one third of deaths in hospitals. Moreover it could be assumed that this specialty is less homogenous than the other four because there is more superspecialisation. Oncologists, hematologists and nephrologists all are internists. Therefore the sample size for internists was set at twice the size of the other specialties. It was attempted to have samples with 70 internists and 35 for each of the other four specialties. This target was almost reached (see Appendix C).

Drawing samples

The sample of general practitioners was drawn from the registry of the Dutch Institute for Primary Health Care (NIVEL). Physicians were selected who had been active in their present practice prior to January 1, 1988. This was done for the sake of some stability in the work situation, which was important for the investigation. A systematic sample was then drawn based on province, and within each province alphabetically according to name. Based on sample fractions, every n-th physician was selected as respondent in each sample. At the same time two additional, spare, samples were drawn according to the same procedure but starting from a different place in the list. A check showed that the initial sample drawn was representative for age, sex and work situation.

The spare samples were used in cases when a respondent refused or did not meet the selection criteria. The selection criterion was that the respondent himself had acted as the treating physician of patients. Moreover, he had to have been active as general practitioner for more than two years. When a respondent refused, the spare sample served to select a respondent who was optimally matched as to age, sex and geographic area. On the other hand, if the respondent did not meet the selection criteria, the first respondent of the spare sample for the particular region was selected, while age and sex of the drop-out were not taken into account.

The sample of nursing home physicians was drawn from the file of the Dutch Association of Nursing Home Physicians (NVVA). This file did not contain information about the period of time someone had worked in a particular institution, so that this criterion, although it of course remained valid, could not be used for advance selection. This file also was set up according to province (using postal codes) and within a province, alphabetically according to name. A systematic sample was drawn thereafter. The replacement procedures for those refusing or for respondents not meeting selection criteria were identical to those applied to the general practitioners.

Specialists were selected from the file of specialists of the office of the Chief Inspector of the Health Supervisory Service. This file is complete but does not contain information as to whether someone is still clinically active. Therefore an age limit (date of birth later than 1924) was set in addition to the requirement that specialisation had to have been completed prior to 1988. Moreover respondents had to be acting as treating physicians of patients admitted to the clinic and had to have been working in the same institution for more than two years – to guarantee some stability in the work situation. The rest of the systematic sample drawing and the replacement procedures were identical to those used for general practitioners.

4.3 Interviewers and appointments

Interviewers

The task of the interviewers was not an easy one, considering the sensitivity of the topic to be investigated, both from an emotional and a legal point of view. It was an absolute condition that a relation of trust had to be established between interviewer and respondent in order to obtain reliable data. Therefore it was decided to use only experienced physicians as interviewers. In addition to some years of experience in a practice these physicians should preferably have completed their studies about 10 years previously. In total 35 interviewers were attracted who each conducted 10 to 15 interviews. Most were invited after personal recommendation by professors of general practice in the various regions. Five of the 35 interviewers were not medically qualified. These non-physicians were included in order to get an impression of the extent to which being a physician would affect the information to be obtained. The five non-physicians, however, had a clear affinity to health care. The interviewers came from places throughout the country, as did the respondents.

The interviewers were asked to study the topic in advance. Moreover, all candidate interviewers underwent two days' training by the Office for Education, Training and Mobility of the University of Amsterdam. At the same time, this training offered the possibility of assessing the suitability of the candidate-interviewers. Several of the candidates were not selected for the study. The training was directed at the substance of the interview as well as the interviewing technique. Special emphasis was put on the making of appointments by telephone calls to the respondents. This telephone call was the first personal contact with the respondent and was therefore crucially important.

Making an appointment

The last step from sampling to appointment is the method of arranging the interview with the respondents.

Respondents and interviewers were matched so that travel times could be kept within reasonable limits. Care was taken that interviewers and respondents did not know each other. The respondents thereafter received a letter stating that they had been included in the sample and that they would be approached by telephone by the interviewer. This letter was accompanied by a letter of recommendation from the Chairman of the Royal Dutch Medical Association and the Chief Inspector of the Health Supervisory Service. The interviewers subsequently telephoned the respondents. If the respondent did not meet the selection criteria, the invitation to participate was cancelled and the interviewer was assigned a new respondent. If the respondent refused, the interviewer enquired as to the motives for this and attempted to clarify possible misunderstandings. If the respondent could not be convinced in this manner, he was still asked to reply to a few questions by telephone. In this way it was attempted to obtain a few characteristics of refusing respondents.

Furthermore, and after obtaining advice from the Royal Dutch Medical Association, it was decided not to compensate the respondents for the time invested in the interview. Occasionally, expenses were paid, e.g. costs of a locum, or compensation for the time needed by an assistant to collect the necessary data.

After respondent and interviewer had made an appointment for the interview, the investigators sent a second letter to the respondent. In addition to a reprint of the paper in the Dutch Journal of Medicine (NTvG) [4] the letter contained a brief questionnaire. The respondent was asked to complete the questionnaire in advance so that the time for the interview could be used as efficiently as possible.

4.4 Questionnaires

The interview was based on two questionnaires, the standard questionnaire and the questionnaire used for the interview. The respondent received the standard questionnaire prior to the interview. This questionnaire contained questions about the most recent (not acute) death for which the respondent had acted as treating physician. The questions in this questionnaire were similar to those in the death certificate study and to those used in the prospective study. This questionnaire is referred to as the standard questionnaire in this book because of its central position in the study. This questionnaire can be found in Appendix A and is discussed in more detail in Chapter 11.

Discussion of the filling-in of the standard questionnaire at the beginning of the interview allowed the possibility of checking the interpretation of the concepts used (see Section 11.3).

After collection and discussion of the standard questionnaire the actual questioning part of the interview started. The questionnaire used contained 120 pages and was thus not added to this book. This questionnaire was developed using several questions from the questionnaire developed by Van der Wal et al. for which the investigators are most grateful.

Seven different types of decisions were then introduced during the interview. Several questions were asked about each of these types of decisions which were, in the order used:

1. Acting on explicit request of the patient (*Chapter 5*).
   The questions concerned requests for euthanasia and assisted suicide. Also, the most recent case of euthanasia or assisted suicide was discussed in more detail.

2. Requests by patients for life-terminating acts that were not acceded to (*Chapter 5*).
   To be able to distinguish clearly between situations that lead, or do not lead to acceding to the request for euthanasia or assisted suicide, attention was given to requests not acceded to.

3. Acting without explicit request of the patient (*Chapter 6*).
   It can also happen, without an explicit request of the patient to terminate life, that a drug is administered that hastens the end of life.

4. Alleviation of pain and symptoms (*Chapter 7*).
   Alleviation of pain and symptoms, particularly with morphine or morphine-like drugs at dosages that could possibly shorten life is an important situation requiring decisions in medical practice. It can be difficult to draw a line between such treatment and euthanasia or performance of life terminating acts without explicit request of the patient.

5. Withdrawing or withholding treatment upon explicit request of the patient (*Section 8.2*).
   This section only covers the situation in which a patient refuses (continuation of) treatment at least partly so as to hasten the end of life.

6. To withdraw or withhold treatment without explicit request of the patient (*Section 8.3*).
   Therapies can also be omitted for reasons other than the patient's request. The case was discussed in greater detail if this happened and life was shortened by more than one month according to the physician.

7. 'Do not resuscitate' decisions (*Section 8.4*).
  This concerns exclusively the anticipatory decision not to attempt resuscitation if cardiac or respiratory arrest occurs.

Following the questions about decisions of this type further questions were asked about the physician's views, with finally a brief evaluation of the interview.

Each serie of questions about the various types of decisions always followed the same pattern. First, questions aimed at quantification were asked: did the respondent ever have to deal with this type of decision and if so, when was the last time and how often had this occurred during the past twelve months? If the respondent had never before been confronted with this situation, he was asked if he would ever be prepared to take this type of decision.

If the respondent had at any time taken a decision of this type, the last relevant case was discussed in greater detail. Questions with respect to this last case then followed, touching on:

- medical aspects;
- social aspects;
- the request of the patient (as far as applicable);
- decision-making by the physician;
- consultations (with colleagues, nurses, patient's relatives);
- carrying-out of the decision;
- completion of the death certificate (natural death or not).

These aspects were covered for almost each type of decision (obviously provided the respondent ever had taken the decision). For certain types of decisions even two cases were subjected to detailed questions. In total, at most ten cases were discussed with each respondent.

Most questions were asked as half open questions; the questionnaire contained a number of categories of possible answers for the benefit of the interviewer. In several cases closed questions were used and the categories of answers for these were offered to the respondent on a card.

After the interview, interviewers were asked to elaborate in their own words on one striking and illustrative example. Information was thus obtained that did justice to the particulars of every decision better than would have been possible by using only the questionnaire.

4.5 From interview to data file

Data protection

The interviews provided an abundance of confidential information. The data were treated in such a way that anonymity of the respondents could be guaranteed. The data obtained from any one respondent could be recognised by means of a number. However, on receipt of the data the original respondent number was replaced by a new number. The relationship between this new number and the original respondent number, i.e. the key, is known only to the investigators. This key will be destroyed upon completion of the study.

In other respects maximal care was also applied to protection of the privacy of respondents and relatives of the deceased and to safeguarding the data. Each interviewer declared in writing that nothing he or she would hear during the interview would ever be repeated outside the framework of the study. All material for the study was handed to the investigators by the interviewers personally. No questionnaires completed during the interview were returned by mail. Data in the data file were filed so that they cannot be used to even indirectly establish a relationship to any individual.

Data file

In order to do justice to all subtle differences occurring in medical practice the investigators reviewed each interview individually with the interviewer. This also served to eliminate uncertainties due to illegible handwriting. If it appeared during this discussion that a certain case was not classified appropriately, this was rectified.

For filing and evaluating data SPSSX (Statistical Package for Social Sciences) was used. All data were introduced twice by different data typists. The two data files were compared as to consistency and any disparities were corrected.

4.6 Response and representativeness

Much attention was devoted to maximising the response. Section 2.6 details the measures taken to obtain maximal cooperation by the medical profession. When appointments were being arranged most intended respondents were immediately prepared to consent to an interview, in spite of having been informed that they had to reserve at least one and a half hours during which they were not to be disturbed.

The intended number of interviews was 410, 150 with general practitioners, 210 with specialists and 50 with nursing home physicians. A total of 599 addresses had to be drawn to reach this number. A total of 23% of the physicians selected for the sample did not meet the selection criteria (see Appendix C). No appointment could be made in 14 cases because of long-lasting illness or because the particular physician could not be located in spite of a thorough search.

A total of 41 physicians, 9% of the number selected, refused to participate in the interviews. Refusal percentages were distributed unevenly over the various categories of physicians. Refusals by general practitioners were 7%, those by specialists 12% and only one of the nursing home physicians refused. A more detailed analysis of the non-responders, reasons for drop-out etc. is presented in Appendix C.

The question of whether those refusing form a select group such that their refusals could lead to serious bias is very important. The refusal percentages were very low, except for the cardiologists and, to a lesser extent, the internists. Moreover, the reasons for refusal varied. Only a very modest bias could result from the total of 15 refusing physicians who stated they were opposed to this study, did not wish to comment or were opposed to euthanasia.

In general there are no reasons to assume that the refusals caused serious bias. It can therefore be concluded that the results of the interview study are valid for Dutch general practitioners, nursing home physicians and the five specialties involved in the study.

4.7 Quality control

Quality control was a major concern:

1. The interviewers were carefully selected and well trained.
2. There was continous intensive contact between investigators and interviewers. All replies from each interview were discussed by one of the investigators with the interviewer. Interviewers had to give their opinion at the end of each interview as to whether the respondent had listened carefully, had given clear and honest replies, etc. Only in one case, in the opinion of both interviewer and investigator, was the information given by the respondent useless. The results of this interview have been deleted from the file. The amount of time required for the interview was sometimes greater than the time available. In such cases parts of the interview were partially or entirely omitted. This only happened a few times and was taken into account in the tables.
3. When interviewing was completed the investigators discussed the overall experiences during interviewing with small groups of interviewers. The interviewers felt that the results of some questions could not be interpreted adequately. These questions were either not considered in this book or were discussed with the appropriate reservations.

Reproducibility

In this type of study it is usually desirable to put the same questions twice to some of the respondents. This gives an impression of the reproducibility of the replies to various questions. However, considering the nature of the interview and the fact that respondents would have to be asked to invest further time in the prospective study, no reproducibility study was carried out.

Validity

The questionnaire for the interviews had been constructed in such a way that the interviewer had to verify in several places that the case under discussion indeed was the case belonging to the correct series of questions. If the case turned out to have been wrongly classified, its classification was rectified either during the interview or subsequently during the review procedure.

To establish validity for the most important questions in the standard questionnaire all respondents were asked to complete prior to the interview the standard questionnaire regarding the most recent non-acute death for which they had been the treating physician. The standard questionnaire was discussed with the physician at the beginning of the interview. In a small number of cases the respondent appeared to have interpreted a question differently from what the investigators had intended or the explanatory comments of the respondent allowed for better interpretation by the investigators (see Section 11.3).

In this connection, a comment can be made about the comparability of the replies of the several professional groups. All specialists and nursing home physicians were interviewed using the same questionnaire. The replies are thus mutually comparable. The general practitioners were interviewed using an earlier version of the questionnaire. There were only minor differences between the two versions. The version intended for the specialists had several questions added about physicians who were still in training and about procedures within the institution. In addition, three questions were improved because the initial formulation could possibly suggest bias. Two questions required profound changes. Thus, except for replies to these five questions, the replies of the general practitioners are also properly comparable to those of the other respondents.

Final opinion

Considering the above we can state that:

– the procedure for selection of the respondents and the low refusal percentage guarantee almost complete representativeness;

- the chance that data of insufficient quality have been included into the data file is virtually nil due to intensive quality control;
- the reproducibility of the replies was not investigated;
- the results will be valid for the most important topics; a reservation must be applied for the data about acting to terminate life without explicit request of the patient. There are several uncertainties regarding this topic (see Chapter 6).

5. Euthanasia and assisted suicide

5.1 Introduction

This chapter contains a discussion of the responses to questions about terminating life upon request of the patient. Starting in Section 5.11 situations are described in which a request of the patient for euthanasia or assisted suicide was refused.

The introduction to this series of questions was:

*I should like to discuss with you euthanasia and assisted suicide. As you probably know, **euthanasia** is defined in The Netherlands as an intentional act to terminate life by a person other than the person involved, upon request of the latter. **Assisted suicide** is defined as the intentional assistance given to a person to terminate his or her own life upon that person's request.*

These are the usual definitions of these forms of terminating life. Using these definitions makes it possible to make links to other investigations which use the

Table 5.1　Respondents who at some time have had a request for euthanasia or assisted suicide and who at some time carried out this request (physician interviews)

	General practitioner n=152 %	Cardio- logist n=34 %	Surgeon n=34 %	Inter- nist n=68 %	Pulmono- logist n=33 %	Neuro- logist n=34 %	Nursing home physician n=50 %	Total n=405 %
Euthanasia or assisted suicide was never discussed	2	38	9	1	6	18	15	5
Euthanasia or assisted suicide "in due course" was requested at some time	92	41	71	85	94	53	53	84
Request "in the foreseeable future" was made at some time	80	50	65	85	85	56	57	76
Euthanasia or assisted suicid carried out at some time	62	18	37	59	56	32	12	54
Euthanasia or assisted suicide carried out within the past 24 months	28	9	21	19	33	24	6	24

Table 5.2   Number of requests for euthanasia or assisted suicide (physician interviews)

	General practitioner n=152	Specialist n=203	Nursing home physician, n=50	total n=405	
Number of requests "in due course"	15700	8950	450	25100	(23400-27000)[1]
Number of requests " in the foreseeable future"	5200	3470	230	8900	(8200-9700)[1]

1) 95% confidence intervals.

same definitions and also to the results of the two part-studies in which the standard form was also used.

5.2 Number of cases

A summary of the most important frequency estimates, subdivided according to medical specialties is presented in Table 5.1. The percentage of respondents indicating that euthanasia or assisted suicide was never discussed between physician and patient is low. Almost all general practitioners and internists have

Table 5.3   Respondents who never carried out euthanasia or assisted suicide (physician interviews)

	General practitioner n=152 %	Cardio-logist n=34 %	Surgeon n=34 %	Internist n=68 %	Pulmono-logist n=33 %	Neuro-logist n=34 %	Nursing home physician n=50 %	Total n=405 %
Ever performed euthanasia or assisted suicide	62	18	37	59	56	32	12	54
Never performed but conceivable	28	44	48	32	28	50	60	34
Would never carry out euthanasia or assisted suicide but would refer	6	15	12	6	9	3	26	8
Would never refer for euthanasia or assisted suicide	3	24	3	3	6	15	2	4
Total	100	100	100	100	100	100	100	100

at some time discussed euthanasia and assisted suicide with one or more of their patients, while 38% of cardiologists indicate that these topics were never discussed between them and their patients.

It also happens that a patient asks that euthanasia or assisted suicide be carried out in due course if suffering becomes unbearable. Most respondents had received such requests in the past. This again relates primarily to general practitioners and internists, but also to pulmonologists, while only 41% of cardiologists answered that they had ever had such a request.

Three quarters of respondents replied affirmatively to the question *"Has it ever happened that a patient explicitly requested euthanasia or assisted suicide within the foreseeable future?"*. The distribution among respondents shows a pattern similar to that for the previous question. Among general practitioners 80% encountered at some time such a request related to the foreseeable future, an average of 71% of the specialists and 57% of nursing home physicians.

A request for euthanasia or assisted suicide was agreed to and carried out at some time by 54% of respondents. There were considerable differences between different kinds of physicians in this respect also. More than half of general practitioners, internists and pulmonologists answered that they had ever agreed to and carried out this kind of request while only a small minority of cardiologists and nursing home physicians (18 and 12% respectively) replied positively. An average of 44% of the specialists have carried out euthanasia or assisted suicide at some time. Moreover it is evident that somewhat fewer than half of the respondents answering that they had at some time agreed to and carried out such a request, had done so at least once during the past 24 months.

Respondents were also asked how often they had performed euthanasia or assisted suicide during the past twelve months and in the preceding twelve months. Based on the data thus obtained one can calculate that, in The Netherlands, euthanasia occurs in 1.9% of all deaths in a particular year. Assisted suicide occurs in 0.3% of all deaths (see Appendix E for the method followed for making these estimates). Based on these data and data from the two part-studies, estimates for the total number of cases of euthanasia and assisted suicide in The Netherlands will be derived in Section 17.3.

Table 5.2 presents estimates (with confidence intervals) of the number of annual requests for euthanasia, both for "in due course" and "in the foreseeable future" with 25 000 and 8900 cases, respectively.

Physicians indicating that they never carried out euthanasia or assisted suicide were asked if they could conceive of situations in which they would be prepared to do so or to refer the patient for this purpose. Table 5.3 shows the replies. No situation in which they would carry out euthanasia or assisted suicide was conceivable for 12% of physicians. The distribution for the various kinds of physicians is comparable to that found for the earlier questions. In a number of cases (8% of all respondents) respondents who will never carry out such an act themselves are prepared to refer patients to a colleague for such a decision. Only 4% of physicians would not be prepared to do this either.

Tables 5.1, 5.2 and 5.3 show convincingly that requests for euthanasia or assisted suicide are part of medical practice for a majority of Dutch physicians who regularly are confronted with terminal patients. It is thus not a question of marginal situations with involvement of a limited number of physicians. The same can be said about carrying out euthanasia or assisted suicide. More than half of the physicians regularly concerned with terminal cases indicated that they themselves have performed euthanasia or assisted suicide.

Almost equally important is the finding that most of the physicians stating that they have never actually performed euthanasia or assisted suicide (see Table 5.3), indicated that they would be prepared to do so under certain circumstances or to refer the patient to a colleague for the purpose. This implies that the great majority of Dutch physicians feel that euthanasia and assisted suicide are actions in which physicians can, under circumstances, collaborate within the framework of their professional actions.

5.3 Characteristics of the patient

In the remainder of this chapter data concerning the most recent case of euthanasia or assisted suicide the respondent has carried out will be used for the description of situations in which decisions are made. This was done because this most recent case was discussed in most detail and, therefore, provides the greatest amount of information. The decision was made to first discuss euthanasia and assisted suicide together and to reserve comparisons between the two for Section 5.10. The reason for this decision was that the number of cases of assisted suicide was so small that it is not always possible to report reliably the appropriate background information. Moreover one can assume that the characteristics of decision-taking will be determined more by the respondent than by the carrying out of euthanasia or assisted suicide.

Euthanasia and assisted suicide are limited here to the administration or supplying or prescribing of drugs. Cases of termination of life by withdrawing treatment are described in Chapter 8.

Table 5.4 shows the distribution of euthanasia and assisted suicide according to age and sex, with the distribution of all deaths in The Netherlands. It is clear that the age distribution of the cases of euthanasia or assisted suicide is different from that of all deaths in The Netherlands. Half of the number of deaths for both sexes falls into the age groups from 20 to 64 years. Relatively far fewer cases of euthanasia or assisted suicide are found in the highest age group.

Table 5.5 shows the distribution among the most important disease groups. In 83% of the most recent death described the patient suffered from cancer. Cancer is the cause of death in 27% of all deaths in The Netherlands. It is clear that this group of diagnoses occupies a special position with respect to euthanasia and assisted suicide.

Finally it can be reported that of the patients who underwent euthanasia or assisted suicide 91% lived independently while 20% were single.

5.4 Medical aspects

It has already been stated in the previous section that the great majority of those requesting euthanasia or assisted suicide were patients suffering from cancer. Table 5.6 shows the aim of the treatment. The respondent could mention more than one aim of treatment. In the majority of cases treatment was palliative (i.e. relief of suffering) or there was no longer any treatment. In several instances life prolonging or curative (i.e. aimed at healing) treatment was given. If the respondent indicated that treatment was therapeutic, treatment of an additional illness was invariably involved, while the most important disease of the patient was untreatable (e.g. pneumonia in a cancer patient).

Table 5.7 summarises possible alternative therapies. The question was: *"Were alternatives available to the treatment given? Here I consider other therapeutic possibilities or possibilities to alleviate pain and/or symptoms"*. In about 80% of cases this question was answered in the negative. In the 20% of cases where there were alternatives in the opinion of the respondent, the question of why the available alternative treatment had not been applied was asked. The reply was almost always that this had been done at the request of the patient.

If in the opinion of the respondent there were no longer any alternatives, it was queried if colleagues had been asked for advice concerning this case. Two thirds of the general practitioners had done so; this figure was 80% for the specialists.

5.5 The request of the patient

Respondents were asked the following question: *"To what extent did the patient make an explicit request?"*. This was always the case. This should not be surprising because the whole series of questions relates to cases in which a request had been made. Table 5.8 shows that in almost all cases a very strong explicit request was involved that was repeated in almost all cases.

The request was always made verbally – except in two cases. In addition, the request was confirmed in writing in 40% of cases. In the opinion of the respondent almost all patients were able to assess their situation and adequately take a decision (98%). There were no patients who were totally incapable of expressing their own will, which obviously was a consequence of the formulation of the introduction.

Concerning the reasons why the patient requested euthanasia or assisted

44

Table 5.4   Age and sex of patients who have undergone euthanasia or assisted suicide, compared
to all deaths in the general population in The Netherlands (physician interviews)

Age	Death through euthanasia or assisted suicide		Total number of deaths in The Netherlands in 1990[1])	
	Males n=95 %	Females n=92 %	Males n=66606 %	Females n=62180 %
	52	49	52	48
0-49	14	22	10	6
50-64	35	29	17	10
65-79	40	36	43	31
80+	11	13	31	53
Total	100	100	100	100

1)   Source: CBS causes-of-death statistics.

Table 5.5   Most important diseases of the patients who have undergone euthanasia or assisted
suicide, compared to all deaths in the general population in The Netherlands
(physician interviews)

	n=187 %	Causes of death (%) in The Netherlands in 1990[1]) n=128786 %
Cancer	83	27
Cardiovascular diseases	4	30
Diseases of the nervous system (incl. stroke)	4	12
Pulmonary diseases	3	8
Mental disorders	1	1
Others (all other categories)	5	22
Total	100	100

1)   Source: CBS causes-of-death statistics.

suicide, it is noteworthy that 'loss of dignity' was mentioned most frequently. In 46% of cases the respondent mentions pain as reason given by the patient. Among these cases ten patients gave pain as the only reason and tiredness of life was the only reason for two requests that life be terminated.

5.6 Arriving at a decision

Table 5.9 shows that the general practitioner consulted a colleague in more than 80% of cases, while in hospital this almost always was the case. The differences are greater with respect to consulting nursing staff. In almost all cases

Table 5.6 **What was the aim of treatment at the time when the decision to perform euthanasia or assisted suicide was made?[1]) (physician interviews)**

	n=187 %
No treatment	14
Only palliative (relief of suffering)	77
Not curative but life prolonging	10
Curative	2

1)   More than one answer could be given to this question.

Table 5.7 **Were there still treatment alternatives[1]) (physician interviews)**

	General practitioner n=91 %	Specialist n=87 %	Total n=184 %
There were alternatives	23	16	21
There were alternatives but patient did not want them	17	16	17
There were no alternatives	77	84	79
Advice asked from colleagues	49	68	55
Total	100	100	100

1)   Nursing home physicians are not mentioned separately but were included in the total.

Table 5.8 **The request of the patient for euthanasia or assisted suicide[1]) (physician interviews)**

	General practitioner n=94 %	Specialist n=87 %	Total n=187 %
Request strongly explicit	97	91	96
Written advance directive present	47	29	43
Request made wholly by patient	99	97	99
Patient totally able to take a decision	99	96	98
Most frequent reason for the request of the patient 2):			
− pain	46	47	46
− loss of dignity	61	46	57
− not dying in a dignified way	47	46	46
− dependence	35	23	33
− tiredness of life	25	16	23

1) Nursing home physicians are not mentioned separately but were included in the total

2) More than one answer could be given to this question.

where nursing of the patient was involved, nurses were consulted in the clinical setting. This was not so in general practice: nurses were involved with the patient in 62% of cases but the general practitioner consulted the nurse in only 41% of these situations.

If the patient had relatives, they were almost always consulted. The lower percentage in the specialist category is largely due to absence of relatives in 9% of cases.

5.7 Performing euthanasia or assisted suicide

Table 5.10 summarises the drugs used for euthanasia or assisted suicide. General practitioners used only morphine in 11% of cases; the percentage of cases in which only morphine was used amounted to 33% for specialists. Almost half of cases received a muscle relaxant in addition to a sedative.

The question of whether performance of euthanasia or assisted suicide was satisfactory technically was answered positively by 83% of respondents.

Table 5.11 summarises the amount of time elapsed between starting the procedure (of euthanasia) and death. In two thirds of cases this was no more than one hour. In a small number of cases it took more than one day.

The question of whether the time elapsed between initiating euthanasia and death was intended in this way was answered positively by three quarters of respondents (Table 5.12). Thirty percent of general practitioners stated that the duration had not been intended in this way. In cases where specialists stated that the duration had not been intended in this way, they were asked whether this meant that it had happened to quickly or too slowly. In most such cases it had apparently lasted too long.

Table 5.13 summarises the answers to the question *"In your opinion, by how long was the life of the patient shortened due to the procedure?"*. In the questionnaire for the general practitioners no distinction had yet been made between the categories 'less than 24 hours' and 'up to one week'.

Among the general practitioners 25% stated that a maximum of one week was involved. This figure was 39% for the specialists. In about one third of cases, life was shortened by more than one month and in 8% of cases by more than half a year. Once more, the reader is cautioned as to the interpretation of data about life shortening (see Section 3.5). Finally respondents were asked if they had had a discussion with relatives after euthanasia had been carried out. Of the general practitioners 91% did and 70% of the specialists.

5.8 Death certificate and reporting

After performing euthanasia or assisted suicide three quarters of the general practitioners and about two thirds of the specialists reported 'natural death' in the

Table 5.9 Consultation concerning euthanasia or assisted suicide with colleagues, nursing staff and relatives[1] (physician interviews)

	General practitioner n=94 %	Specialist n=87 %	Total n=187 %
Consultation with colleagues	81	93	84
Nursing staff involved with patient	62	94	70
Consultation with nursing staff if involved with patient	*41*	*96*	*60*
Consultation with relatives	97	85	94

1) Nursing home physicians are not mentioned separately but were included in the total.

Table 5.10 Drugs used for euthanasia or assisted suicide[1] (physician interviews)

	General practitioner n=94 %	Specialist n=87 %	Total n=187 %
Sedatives only (excl. morphine)[2]	20	15	19
Sedatives + muscle relaxants[3]	50	38	47
Morphine only	11	22	13
Morphine in combination with other drugs (excl. muscle relaxants)	13	16	13
Other drugs and combinations	6	11	7
Total	100	100	100

1) Nursing home physicians are not mentioned separately but were included in the total.
2) Drugs reducing consciousness, such as benzodiazepines and barbiturates.
3) Curare-like agents.

Table 5.11 Time elapsed between starting euthanasia or assisted suicide until death[1] (physician interviews)

	General practitioner n=94 %	Specialist n=86 %	Total n=186 %
1 minute or less	6	–	5
1 – 10 minutes	32	18	28
10 minutes – 1 hour	28	42	32
1 hour – 1 day	28	28	28
1 day – 1 week	6	12	7
1 – 4 weeks	1	–	1
Total	100	100	100

1) Nursing home physicians are not mentioned separately but were included in the total.

declaration of death (Table 5.14). Of the six cases reported by nursing home physicians, however, only one cause of death was reported as natural. The most important reasons for declaring natural death were: the 'fuss' of a legal investigation (55%), fear of prosecution (25%), the desire to safeguard relatives from a judicial enquiry (52%) and bad experiences in the past with stating non-natural death (12%). Moreover it should be reported as remarkable that 8 general practitioners and 15 specialists declared that in spite of euthanasia or assisted suicide they had experienced the patient's death as a natural one.

When no declaration of natural death was made, the coroner was contacted in 60% of the cases, police in some 40% and the public prosecutor in some 40%. The inspector of health was contacted in only a small minority of cases. It is noteworthy that general practitioners contact police much more often than do the specialists. The specialist more often contacts the public prosecutor.

5.9 Rules of due care

Respondents were asked a great number of questions with the purpose of detecting to what extent they had adhered to the rules of due care with respect to euthanasia and assisted suicide (see also Section 9.2). The replies to the relevant questions are shown in table 5.15.

The table shows that in nearly all cases there was a voluntarily made request of the patient for euthanasia or assisted suicide. It can also be stated that in nearly all cases a long-lasting and carefully considered desire to die is involved, considering the large percentage of repeated requests and also the large percentage of patients who have a good understanding of their illness and prognosis.

In almost 80% of cases there were no therapeutic alternatives for the patient. When these did exist, the respondent did not apply these because in almost all instances the patient did not give permission. A colleague was consulted in 84% of cases, as has been discussed in Section 5.6.

One of the strict rules of due care proposed by the Cabinet in 1987 is that relatives of the patient must be informed, unless the patient does not want this. Table 5.15 shows that this rule was followed in almost all cases.

The rule about recording the decision making process was less well adhered to. Somewhat more than one half of the general practitioners and three quarters of the specialists kept adequate records.

5.10 Euthanasia compared with assisted suicide

If one distinguishes euthanasia and assisted suicide mainly by emphasising the person who administers the drug, there is, in principle, a clear distinction. For the analysis a death was classified on the basis of the person administering the last

49

Table 5.12 Was the time elapsed between initiating euthanasia and death as intended?[1] (physician interviews)

	General practitioner n=94 %	Specialist n=86 %	Total n=186 %
Yes	70	86	74
No, too fast		1	
No, too slow		13	
No[2]	30		26
Total	100	100	100

1) The nursing home physicians are not mentioned separately but were included in the total.
2) For general practitioners no difference was made between too fast and too slow.

Table 5.13 Extent of shortening of life by euthanasia or assisted suicide[1] (physician interviews)

	General practitioner n=92 %	Specialist n=85 %	Total n=183 %
No shortening	1	–	1
Less than 24 hours[2]		–	
Up to one week	24	39	28
1 to 4 weeks	47	29	42
1 to 6 months	20	24	21
More than half a year	9	6	8
Total	100	100	100

1) Nursing home physicians are not mentioned separately but were included in the total.
2) General practitioners only had 'up to one week' as a possible answer. No difference was thus made in their cases between 'less than 24 hours' and 'up to one week'.

Table 5.14 Death certificate in case of euthanasia or assisted suicide[1] (physician interviews)

	General practitioner n=93 %	Specialist n=85 %	Total n=184 %
No declaration of natural death made	25	35	28
In that case contact set up with[2]:			
– municipal coroner	65	45	60
– police	57	10	42
– public prosecutor	35	62	42
– inspector of health	9	4	8
Declaration of natural death made	75	65	72
Total	100	100	100

1) Nursing home physicians are not mentioned separately but were included in the total.
2) More than one answer could be given to this question.

drug, either as assisted suicide (if the patient himself takes the drug) or as euthanasia (if someone else, the physician included, administers the drug). This distinction was however not applied in the sections above. The most recent case treated by the respondent was used in the tables, regardless of whether it involved euthanasia or assisted suicide. If a respondent had ever performed both euthanasia and assisted suicide, the most recent occurrence for each of these acts was questioned in detail. This section discusses this information. Thus the data concern a larger number of cases, i.e. 160 cases of euthanasia and 41 cases of assisted suicide.

Deceased who had undergone euthanasia differ in several ways from those who had received assistance with suicide. The percentage of males was 48% for euthanasia and 68% for assisted suicide. There was, however, almost no age difference: 49% of the patients euthanised were were younger than 65 years of age, while this percentage was 51% for assisted suicide.

It is noteworthy that, of the most important illnesses, cancer was the most important disease in about the same percentages of cases of euthanasia and

Table 5.15   To what extent were the rules of due care with respect to euthanasia or assisted suicide strictly adhered to?[1] (physician interviews)

	General practitioner n=94 %	Specialist n=87 %	Total n=187 %
Request of the patient			
– explicit request	97	91	96
– request made wholly by the patient	99	97	99
– repeated request	94	94	94
– patient had good insight into disease and prognosis	100	99	100
Alternatives			
– no alternatives	77	84	79
– alternatives but patient no longer wanted them	17	16	17
Consultations			
– consult with colleagues	81	93	84
– relatives informed	97	85	94
– relatives not informed because there were none	–	9	2
– relatives not informed because patient did not want this	2	1	2
– relatives not informed for other reasons	1	5	2
Records			
– written records kept	54	74	60

1) Nursing home physicians are not mentioned separately but were included in the total.

Table 5.16   Did you ever not accede to a request for euthanasia or assisted suicide? (physician interviews)

	General practitioner n=151 %	Specialist n=200 %	Nursing Home Physician n=50 %	Total n=401 %
Ever not acceded to a serious request	44	46	46	44
Request not acceded to during the past 24 months	30	29	29	30

assisted suicide: 82% and 83% respectively. Considering the other groups of diseases it is to be noted that only 2 of the 41 patients who were assisted with suicide suffered from a psychiatric disease. This diagnosis did not appear in the euthanasia group.

Euthanasia and assisted suicide differ somewhat with respect to shortening life: for euthanasia shortening life by more than one half year occurred in 5% of cases, while this percentage was 15% for assisted suicide.

5.11 Refused requests for euthanasia and assisted suicide

Previous sections concerned situations in which the request of the patient was acceded to. Requests not acceded to by the physician will be considered in this section.

In the interview this topic was introduced as follows:

In this study we also want to get an impression of situations in which the patient requests euthanasia or assisted suicide but in which the physician decides not to accede to this request. Obviously there is a difference between a situation in which the patient indicates that in due course he will possibly make a request and the situation in which the patient makes a explicit request for euthanasia or assisted suicide to be carried out now or in the foreseeable future.

The questions only refer to requests 'in the foreseeable future'. The first question therefore was: *"Has it happened that a patient asked for euthanasia or assisted suicide in the foreseeable future but that you decided not to accede to this request? It would have to be a request that you took seriously but that you nevertheless did not accede to."*

Such a request was not acceded to at some time by 44% of all respondents (see table 5.16). The agreement between the different kinds of physicians (general practitioners, specialists and nursing home physicians) was noteworthy. This was also true for the percentage of physicians who declined at least once to accede to such a request within the past two years: this was about one third for each type of physician.

Based on the total of answers received we estimate that the total number of requests seriously considered but refused amounts to 4000 per annum in The Netherlands. If this figure is compared to the total number of requests for euthanasia or assisted suicide within the foreseeable future and the total number of requests that have been agreed to, there still are some 2000 requests that have not been categorised. The following explanations can be considered, apart from the confidence intervals around the estimates:

— some patients died before the request could be acceded to;
— some requests were not considered as explicit by the physician;
— some requests were not really refused but the request was also not followed up because the patient changed his mind.

Comparison of Table 5.16 with Table 5.1 shows that the percentage of respondents who indicate ever having performed euthanasia or assisted suicide is greater than the percentage indicating ever having refused a serious request. The most obvious explanation is that if the physician is not prepared to accede to a request for euthanasia or assisted suicide the development of an explicit request that has to be refused very explicitly, is somehow prevented.

The most recent cases described by the physicians were used for the description of the requests not acceded to.

Table 5.17 shows the distribution among the most important groups of diseases. The diagnosis was cancer in 56% of the cases. The second most important group was that of mental disorders with 14%. These percentages differ from the percentages for the cases accepted, where the percentage of patients with cancer was 78%.

The age distribution of males did not differ from that found for the cases where the request had been accepted. The females whose request was refused were older, on the average, than those whose request was accepted. Also, there were relatively more males than females whose requests had been refused (55% versus 45%).

In two thirds of the cases the request of the patient had been explicit and strong (see Table 5.18). This is less than in the case of accepted requests for euthanasia or assisted suicide, where the request was practically always explicit. One fifth of the patients had a written advance directive concerning life termination.

About one third of the patients were unable or not totally able to assess their situation and thus to take a decision adequately on this basis. The most

Table 5.17 **Most important diseases of patients whose requests for euthanasia or assisted suicide were not acceded to (physician interviews)**

	n=176 %
Cancer	56
Cardiovascular diseases	7
Diseases of the nervous system (incl. stroke)	10
Pulmonary diseases	4
Mental disorders	14
Others (all other categories)	10
Total	100

Table 5.18 **The refused request of the patient for euthanasia or assisted suicide and the degree of (in)ability to take a decision (physician interviews)**

	General practitioner n=66 %	Specialist n=87 %	Nursing home physician n=23 %	Total n=176 %
Strongly explicit request	58	77	61	63
Written advance directive available	18	19	22	19
Patient able to assess the situation and take a decision adequately?				
– totally able	67	61	65	65
– not totally able	26	34	31	28
– totally unable	8	5	4	7
Most important cause for not being (totally) able[1]:				
– *emotionally too labile*	36	44	38	39
– *mental disorder*	27	25	25	27

1)   More than one answer could be given to this question.

Table 5.19 **Consultation with others than the patient in cases for which a request was not acceded to (physician interviews)**

	General practitioner n=66 %	Specialist n=87 %	Nursing home physician n=23 %	Total n=176 %
Colleague consulted	41	56	44	45
Nurse consulted	5	38	57	18
Partner of patient consulted	18	14	9	16
(Other) relatives consulted	15	10	35	15
Religious or spiritual adviser consulted	3	5	22	5

frequently cited reason for being (partly) unable to take a decision was that in the opinion of the physician the patient was too instable emotionally or was psychically disturbed.

A colleague was consulted in slightly less than half the cases before it was decided not to accept the request. Nurses or relatives were consulted in only a small number of cases (Table 5.19).

The physician's reasons for not accepting the patient's request varied widely (see Table 5.20). In one third of the cases the physician felt that there were still other treatment possibilities for the patient, including further possibilities of alleviation of pain and/or symptoms. In 20% of the cases, respondents felt that the patient's request had not been properly considered. It should be mentioned that it was precisely the strong manner in which the patient made a request that led some respondents to feel that the request had not been considered properly. In 24% of the cases the physician felt that there was poor understanding of the disease. In 26% the physician indicated that, in general, he was prepared to perform euthanasia or assisted suicide but had objections in this particular case. Another 19% of respondents objected to euthanasia or assisted suicide in general. This percentage does not completely agree with the percentage of respondents stating that they cannot imagine any situation in which they would be prepared to perform euthanasia or assisted suicide (Table 5.3). This difference is understandable in view of the different formulation of the two questions. The question described in Table 5.1 was: *"Can you conceive of situations in which*

Table 5.20   Most important considerations for not acceding to a request for euthanasia or assisted suicide[1] (physician interviews)

	General practitioner n=66 %	Specialist n=87 %	Nursing home physician n=23 %	Total n=176 %
There still were alternatives (incl. possibilities of alleviation of pain and/or symptoms)	29	45	26	33
Suffering was not unbearable	11	8	9	10
Request was not well considered	23	15	17	20
Patient did not have proper understanding of his disease	21	29	22	24
Patient withdrew request after thorough discussion	5	6	17	6
Physician had objections in this particular case	27	23	30	26
General objection by physician to euthanasia and/or assisted suicide	20	18	22	19

1)   More than one answer could be given to this question.

you would perform euthanasia or assisted suicide?'' The answer that the respondent could consider doing this under unusual circumstances does not mean that the physician would not have objections to euthanasia or assisted suicide in general.

6. Life-terminating acts without the patient's explicit request

6.1 Introduction

Life-terminating acts by a physician without the patient's explicit request are discussed in this chapter. The series of questions formulated for this type of action was directed towards situations which should be comparable in all respects with those discussed in Chapter 5 (euthanasia and assisted suicide), except with respect to the patient's request. The introduction to this series of questions was as follows:

There are situations in which it is decided to perform a life-terminating act without the patient's request to do so. This can occur if the patient had made only vague remarks but not an explicit request. Other situations in which this might happen are, e.g., those in which the patient is no longer able to make such a request, or if the condition of the patient is evidently intolerable.

The interviewer was instructed to consider as acts the administration of drugs but not acts such as for example withdrawing artificial respiration. The latter would be discussed in another series of questions. In addition, the interviewer was given the following instruction:

The respondent determines what is a non-explicit request. A situation may be involved in which absolutely no request was made or it may be a situation in which the patient made a request, but not explicitly so.

In this introduction and the instruction to the interviewer it was not specified as a constraint that the cases involved must be cases in which the explicit purpose was hastening of the end of life. This means that the comparability of the actions discussed here to the actions discussed in Chapter 5 is not guaranteed. Furthermore, no question was included concerning the intention of the physician. This complicates the interpretation of the results.

The replies to the question and the relevant cases discussed suggest that some of the respondents interpreted the description given above much more broadly than the investigators had intended. This latter group of respondents indicated that they have performed a life-terminating act without explicit request of the patient more than once in the past twelve months. The examples discussed always deal with the intensification of alleviation of pain and/or symptoms in patients in the last phase of their disease. An example could be the history of a female demented nursing home patient who suffered so much pain from bedsores that morphine was necessary. She very rapidly required increasing doses of morphine and died five days after the initiation of morphine administration. This type of case belongs, in principle, to Chapter 7: Alleviation of pain and symptoms.

Due to the widely varying interpretation of these questions and to the absence of the question as to the intent of the physician, the number of cases of life-terminating acts without explicit request of the patient cannot be reliably estimated on the basis of interview data. The remainder of this chapter concerns the characteristics of the most recent cases described by the respondents. Interpretation of these results will follow in Section 6.9.

The remaining cases presented by the respondents can be divided into two types of situations in which a decision had to be taken.

First, there are a number of cases in which the patient who has become unable to make a decision had expressed earlier the wish to have life terminated. This relates to comments such as ''if I cannot be saved any more, you must give me something'' or ''doctor, please don't let me suffer for too long''. In such cases the earlier request of the patient was acted upon. Requests of this type were mentioned in 28% of the cases discussed here. They clearly are a transition to the type of situation discussed in Chapter 5.

Table 6.1   Respondents who at some time performed a life-terminating act without explicit request of the patient (physician interviews)

	General practitioner n=151 %	Specialist n=195 %	Nursing home physician n=49 %	Total n=395 %
Performed a life-terminating act at some time without explicit request	30	25	10	27
Performed a life-terminating act without explicit request within the past 24 months	9	16	2	10
Acting without explicit request conceivable	32	31	27	32
Would never act thus without explicit request	38	44	63	41
Total	100	100	100	100

Another group of cases refers to patients in the final stage of their disease who deteriorate unexpectedly rapidly and where proper discussion between patient and physician no longer is possible. Further study of such cases shows that this concerns situations where the patient is terminal and the physician decides not to prolong suffering. An example may be a dying patient suffering from non-specific respiratory disease whose shortness of breath can no longer be relieved and where the physician decides 'not to needlessly prolong suffering'; or a patient dying of cancer with reduced consciousness who suffers such pain due to brain metastases that a life-terminating act appears to be the only solution considering the degrading situation. In such cases extensive discussion with the patient is impossible and the patient could, considering the seriousness of the disease, not be considered to be able to reach a decision adequately.

The cases described by respondents cannot all be assigned to one of the above categories. These three types of decision-making situations cannot be distinguished sharply. A respondent sometimes indicated that greater involvement of patient and others in the decision-making process would certainly have been possible. Several times cases were involved that had occurred several years ago and the respondent indicated that due to present day acceptance of clear decision-making in such matters he certainly would now have opted for a more extensive decision-making process.

6.2   Occurrence of life-terminating acts without explicit request of the patient

Table 6.1 presents an overview of life-terminating acts without explicit request of the patient. Of the total number of all physicians interviewed 27% said they had done this at some time. This percentage was considerably lower, i.e. 10%, for nursing home physicians. As 'at some time' could mean 'a long time ago' it was important to know how many physicians had acted in this manner fairly recently (in the past 24 months). Of all physicians, 10% acted without explicit request during the past 24 months; the differences between types of physicians were large: 9% of general practitioners, 16% of specialists and one physician of the group of nursing home physicians (2%).

In addition to the 27% of respondents saying they had performed a life-terminating act without explicit request of the patient at some time, 32% indicated that they could conceive of situations when they would decide on life-terminating acts without explicit request of the patient, while 41% considered such a situation inconceivable. Table 6.1 shows that more than half of the physicians either have performed a life-terminating act without request or can imagine a situation in which they would act thus. This means that this MDEL also is an important topic for many physicians.

Table 6.2   Age and sex of deceased where life-terminating acts were performed without explicit request, compared to all deaths in the general population in The Netherlands (physician interviews)

Age	Deaths due to a life-terminating act without explicit request		Total number of deaths in The Netherlands in 1990[1])	
	Males n=58 %	Females n=37 %	Males n=66606 %	Females n=62180 %
	58	42	52	48
0 – 49	10	11	10	6
50 – 64	28	22	17	10
65 – 79	49	29	43	31
80+	13	38	31	53
Total	100	100	100	100

1)   Source: CBS causes-of death statistics.

Table 6.3   Most important diseases of patients on which life- terminating acts were performed without explicit request, compared to all deaths in the general population in The Netherlands (physician interviews)

	n=96 %	Distribution of death causes in The Netherlands in 1990[1]) n=128786 %
Cancer	70	27
Cardiovascular diseases	3	30
Diseases of the nervous system (incl. stroke)	9	12
Pulmonary diseases	3	8
Mental disorders	3	1
Others (all other categories)	12	22
Total	100	100

1)   Source: CBS causes-of-death statistics.

6.3 Patient characteristics

In the interview a description was asked of the last time a life terminating act that was performed without explicit request. The percentages in the tables all refer to the most recent case. 'Acting' has been limited here to administering drugs and does not concern withdrawing treatment.

Table 6.2 shows the age and sex distribution. Two thirds of the deceased were over 65 years of age. Thus, this group was younger on the average than could have been expected on the basis of the age distribution of all deceased taken together, but was older than the group of those dying due to euthanasia or assisted suicide. These age differences indicate that performing a life-terminating act without explicit request occurs on the average with older patients than does euthanasia or assisted suicide.

Table 6.3 presents the distribution of the most frequently occurring diseases groups. 70% of the patients suffered from cancer. Thus, this illness also occurs relatively frequently in these patients as compared to all deaths in The Netherlands.

Table 6.4 presents information about the patient's ability to express his/her own wish. As pointed out in Chapter 3, ability to express his/her own wish is defined as "being able to assess the situation and then take a decision adequately". Of the patients, 86% were not (totally) able to do so. The cause of this was, in 54% of these cases, reduced consciousness. One out of three of such patients was permanently unconscious (amongst whom only a few who were in a persistent vegatative state).

6.4 Medical aspects

In replying to the question as to the aim of the treatment, 87% of the respondents replied that this was palliative (relief of suffering) only, or that there was no treatment at all. There was still a curative element (aimed at a cure) in 7% of the cases. However, it should be said that aiming at a cure does not imply that this was successful. An example is a cancer patient who had a serious

Table 6.4 Degree of ability of patients to take a decision in cases where life was terminated without the patient's explicit request[1] (physician interviews)

	General practitioner n=45 %	Specialist n=47 %	Total n=97 %
Patient able to assess the situation and take a decision adequately			
− totally able	16	9	14
− not totally able	9	17	11
− totally unable	76	74	75
Most important cause for not being (totally) able[2]			
− reduced consciousness	50	65	54
− permanently unconscious	34	25	31
− demented	5	6	8

1) Nursing home physicians are not mentioned separately but were included in the total.

2) More than one answer could be given to this question.

62

Table 6.5 Medical aspects of patients in whom a life-terminating act was performed without explicit request of the patient[1]) (physician interviews)

	General practitioner n=45 %	Specialist n=47 %	Total n=97 %
There were alternatives	7	11	8
There were no alternatives	93	89	92
Morphine or morphine-like drugs were required	84	52	76
Morphine or morphine-like drugs were required but were not effective against pain and/or symptoms	52	27	45

1) Nursing home physicians are not mentioned separately but were included in the total.

cerebral haemorrhage that led to untreatable epileptic fits. The reply that treatment was aimed at cure was based on cancer chemotherapy. However, the patient did not respond to this therapy. In all eleven cases in which the reply was 'curative', the purpose of the therapy was nullified by a new complication or was not reached.

Table 6.5 shows that there were still treatment alternatives in 8% of cases in which a life-terminating act was performed without explicit request of the patient. These alternatives were not used by the physician because the patient had indicated no longer wanting this (four times), because "it only would prolong suffering" (three times) or because the gain to be expected was no longer in due proportion to the treatment (three times).

Table 6.5 also shows several important data concerning other medical aspects which are of great significance for a correct interpretation of these cases. The respondents were asked if morphine or morphine-like drugs were administered as part of the alleviation of pain and/or symptoms. This was done in three quarters of the cases. Moreover, in spite of these drugs, pain or other symptoms could not be treated adequately in 45% of the cases. On one hand this attests to the seriousness of suffering in the situations described and on the other hand it exemplifies the difficulty of distinguishing these cases from those described in the next chapter under "alleviation of pain and symptoms".

6.5 Previous wishes of the patient

The respondents were asked the following question: *"Had the patient ever indicated anything about termination of life?"* Table 6.6 shows that this happened in 28% of cases. The request that life be terminated was not made explicitly but the patient indicated that "this is no longer necessary" or asks "Doctor, please help, I no longer want to suffer".

Somewhat fewer than three quarters of the patients did not indicate anything but were no longer able to do this at the moment of action. Answering the question as to why terminating life had not been discussed with the patient, it almost always was stated that this was no longer possible. There was a written advance directive about life termination in two cases. These cases could therefore be considered as euthanasia.

The reply to the question as to who had raised the topic of termination of life was 'no one' in one third of the cases. In about one half of the cases relatives raised the issue. For general practitioners this distribution differs from that for specialists. In hospital, nursing staff or a colleague took the initiative to discuss termination of life with the (treating) physician in more than 50% of cases.

The low percentage of patients that, according to the respondent, raised the issue of termination of life is remarkable when it is compared to the percentage of patients who had at some time given indications regarding this issue. The latter is apparently not considered as an initiative. Alternatively, something may not have been indicated to the physician but for instance, to relatives.

6.6 Arriving at a decision

The respondent was then asked what had been the most important considerations for his decision. Table 6.7 summarises the replies.

The replies give a clear picture. Suffering, the patient's pain or the low quality of life are mentioned in 30% of cases. In almost two thirds of cases the physician stated that there was no prospect of improvement of the situation; in 39% the

Table 6.6   Previously expressed wishes by the patient with respect to life termination and the person raising this topic[1]) (physician interviews)

	General practitioner n=45 %	Specialist n=46 %	Total n=96 %
Patient indicated something about terminating life at some time	29	24	28
Written advance directive available	2	0	2
Who raised the topic of terminating life with you?[2])			
– no one	32	39	34
– colleague	2	25	8
– patient	–	6	2
– nurse	2	29	9
– relatives	57	16	47
– others	9	2	7

1)   Nursing home physicians are not mentioned separately but were included in the total.

2)   More than one answer could be given to this question.

respondent felt that any further medical therapy was futile and in 33% that suffering should not be prolonged unnecessarily.

It should not be surprising that the patient's wish is mentioned in 17% of cases while the patient had given some indication about terminating life in 28% of cases (Table 6.6). The question as to the physician's reasons was phrased as an open question. It was very important to the physicians whether they could really appreciate the wish of the patient. As to the physician's reason for the decision, it was not so much the wish of the patient, but the circumstances that made the physician appreciate the patient's wish.

It also is of importance to state that economic considerations hardly ever

Table 6.7 **The most important considerations by the physician to perform a life-terminating act without explicit request of the patient[1] [2] (physician interviews)**

	General practitioner n=45 %	Specialist n=47 %	Total n=97 %
Wish by patient	20	8	17
Pain/suffering of patient	33	21	30
Low quality of life	31	26	31
No chance of improvement	62	54	60
All medical therapy had become futile	36	54	39
A therapy had been withdrawn but patient did not die	2	7	3
No needless prolongation	33	32	33
Relatives could no longer cope	40	7	32
Economic considerations (e.g. scarcity of beds)	–	2	1
Other	–	2	1

1) Nursing home physicians are not mentioned separately but were included in the total.

2) More than one answer could be given to this question.

Tabel 6.8 **Consultation with colleagues, nursing staff and relatives about performing a life-terminating act without explicit request of the patient[1] (physician interviews)**

	General practitioner n=45 %	Specialist n=47 %	Total n=97 %
Consultation with colleagues	40	71	48
Nursing staff involved with patient	77	100	84
Consultation with nursing staff (if involved with patient)	44	98	62
Consultation with relatives	78	55	72

1) Nursing home physicians are not mentioned separately but were included in the total.

played a role. This reason was mentioned only once by a specialist, in combination with several other considerations.

Table 6.8 shows that a colleague has been consulted in almost one half of the cases (general practitioners: 40%, specialists: 71%). If nursing staff were involved with the patient (this is always the case in hospitals or nursing homes), they were consulted in 60% of cases. Relatives were consulted in more than 70% of cases.

For cases of euthanasia or assisted suicide colleagues, nursing staff and relatives were consulted in 84%, 60% and 94% of cases, respectively. Thus, in the situations described here colleagues were consulted less often. The reason mentioned for not having done so was, in 68% of the cases, that the physician felt no need for consultation because the situation had been clear. This fact should also be considered in the light of the very brief period by which life was shortened (Table 6.10).

6.7 Performing the act

Table 6.9 summarises the drugs used. In 44% of cases the end of life had been hastened only by means of morphine. This had happened in only 13% of cases of euthanasia or assisted suicide. Muscle relaxants were used for euthanasia or assisted suicide more than twice as often as when life was terminated without explicit request. The frequent use of morphine again demonstrates that the difference from alleviation of pain or symptoms (Chapter 7) is far from sharp.

Table 6.10 shows the distribution of the periods by which life was shortened. The end of life was hastened by a maximum of one week in 71% of cases. This fraction was 29% for euthanasia.

6.8 The death certificate

The death certificate almost always states that the patient died a natural death. Only one general practitioner reported a non-natural death to the public prosecutor. In this case the public prosecutor decided not to prosecute. The most important reasons to record a natural death are the 'fuss' of a judicial investigation (47%), the view that the death was in fact natural (43%) and the desire to safeguard relatives from a judicial enquiry (28%).

6.9 Discussion

This section presents a brief review of the results described in this chapter.

The data obtained in this part of the interview do not provide a sufficient basis for a reliable quantitative estimate. The most important reason is the

Table 6.9   **Drugs used to terminate life without explicit request of the patient[1]) (physician interviews)**

	General practitioner n=45 %	Specialist n=47 %	Total n=97 %
Sedating drugs only (excl. morphine)[2])	7	23	11
Sedating drugs + muscle relaxants[3])	22	13	19
Morphine only	49	31	44
Morphine in combination with other drugs (excl.muscle relaxants)	18	17	18
Other drugs and combinations	4	17	8
Total	100	100	100

1)   Nursing home physicians are not mentioned separately but were included in the total.
2)   Drugs reducing consciousness, such as benzodiazepines and barbiturates.
3)   Curare-like drugs.

Table 6.10   **Extent of shortening of life due to performing a life-terminating act without explicit request of the patient[1]) (physician interviews)**

	General practitioner n=45 %	Specialist n=47 %	Total n=97 %
No shortening	4	2	4
Less than 24 hours[2])		33	} 67
Up to one week	71	27	
1 to 4 weeks	18	27	21
1 to 6 months	7	8	7
More than half a year	–	2	1
Total	100	100	100

1)   Nursing home physicians are not mentioned separately but were included in the total.
2)   General practitioners only had 'up to one week' as a possible answer. No difference was thus made in their cases between 'less than 24 hours' and 'up to one week'.

respondents' rather differing interpretation of the series of questions asked. Some mentioned situations in which decisions had to be made that primarily related to alleviation of pain and symptoms and that are discussed in Chapter 7. When questioned about alleviation of pain and symptoms these respondents often indicated already having answered these questions when discussing acts to terminate life without explicit request of the patient. Other physicians had interpreted these questions as referring to an extremely momentous decision. This can be concluded from the fact that 41% of respondents said that no situations are imaginable in which they would decide to perform a life-terminating act without explicit request of the patient. Due to the absence of a question as to the physician's intent in this part of the interview one cannot distinguish clearly between the physicians' various interpretations of these questions.

The statistical distributions reported in this chapter agree in many respects with those of the chapter describing alleviation of pain and symptoms (Chapter 7). For instance, the distributions of age, sex and most important diseases are almost identical in the two chapters. The estimated amount of time by which life was shortened is almost the same in both chapters, while it was much greater when euthanasia or assisted suicide was performed.

The situations discussed in this chapter also differ in several other aspects from those described in the previous chapter (on euthanasia and assisted suicide). The drugs administered, e.g., were much more often morphine only, in combination with, or without other sedatives and less often sedatives together with muscle relaxants than had been reported for euthanasia. (Administering sedation, followed by muscle relaxants, is the method of choice to terminate life in The Netherlands in a patient who is not yet in the terminal phase). Also the time course between administering the drug and the death of the patient was longer on the average than in the case of euthanasia or assisted suicide. Moreover, life had been shortened by a maximum of one week in 71% of cases and by more than half a year in only one of 97 cases.

This information confirms the suspicion that there is an important borderline area between euthanasia and performing a life-terminating act without request on one hand and on the other hand between performing a life-terminating act without request and intensifying alleviation of pain and symptoms. This borderline area is discussed in more detail in Chapter 17.

Figure 6.1 further reviews the distribution of the 97 cases with respect to several important characteristics. The numbers shown in the figure were not weighted, i.e. the numbers were not increased to values representative for The Netherlands. In 13 of the 97 cases the physician discussed it with the patient but there had been no explicit request. In 69 of the 84 cases in which there had been no discussion, the patient was totally unable to assess the situation and to take a decision adequately. In nine cases the patient was not totally able to do so, while the patient was totally able to do so in six cases. Of these six patients that apparently had been considered as totally able to take a decision, four had given some indication in the past while two had not done this.

In both cases this involved patients treated by general practitioners. The cases dated from the early 1980s. The first case was a patient with a lung tumor with metastases who suffered much pain. The physician had known this patient for 15 years. The most important consideration for the physician to administer an overdose of morphine was to no longer prolong suffering. The case had not been discussed with a colleague ''because at that time general practitioners worked

Figure 6.1 Performing a life-terminating act without explicit request by the patient (numbers not weighted) (physician interviews)

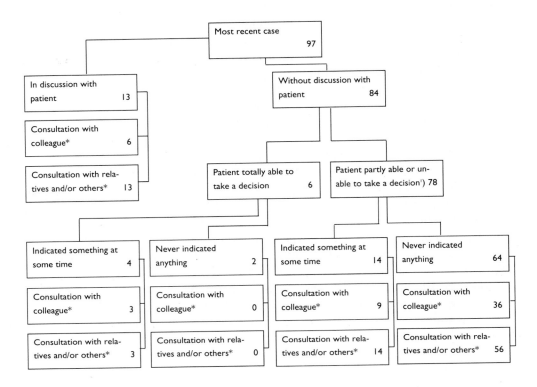

1) 78 patients, 9 of whom were partially unable and 69 totally unable to take a decision.
*) 'Consultation with a colleague' and 'Consultation with relatives and/or others' can occur in combination.

much more independently". In a non-verbal understanding with the patient's wife the decision to increase greatly the dose of morphine was taken.

The second, comparable case also concerned a patient with cancer in whom alleviation of pain and/or symptoms was intensified to the extent that the patient died within one day. "The patient's suffering was intolerable for everyone. Patient and relatives could no longer stand it." The respondent was one of those indicating that under present day circumstances with increased openness around these problems, he probably would have initiated more extensive consultations.

Within the group of 64 patients who were (partly) unable to take a decision and with whom no discussion had taken place there were five cases in which no consultation with others (relatives, colleagues) had taken place. Four of these five deceased were patients who suffered seriously and in whom life was shortened by at most a few hours or days. In one case it was a seriously ill patient whose life, in the opinion of the physician, may have been shortened by one to four weeks.

6.10 Conclusions

In summary, the following conclusions can be drawn:

1. Acting to terminate life without explicit request of the patient occurs in The Netherlands.
2. Some cases fit into the borderline area between euthanasia and acts to terminate life without explicit request of the patient, others fit into the borderline area between the latter category and that in which alleviation of pain and symptoms with morphine was undertaken using doses that almost certainly would shorten life.
3. Although the acts to terminate life discussed in this chapter occurred without explicit request of the patient, about one quarter of the number of patients had previously indicated something regarding life termination.
4. Almost all cases involved seriously ill and dying patients who clearly suffered severely and were no longer able to take a decision.
5. In the interview, two cases of life-terminating acts were described in which the patient had never indicated anything, but in which the patient had been totally able to take a decision. These were cases that had occurred a long time ago.
6. The interviews yielded five cases of life-terminating acts in which discussion with the patient was no longer possible and in which the patient had never indicated anything, and no consultation with others had taken place. Four of these cases involved dying patients who suffered severely and in whom life was shortened by several hours or days at most.
7. One case was found in which the physician performed a life-terminating act without explicit request of the patient, where discussing with the patient was not possible and where life was shortened by more than six months. In the opinion of the physician the patient obviously had not yet reached the terminal phase of the disease.

Life-terminating acts without explicit request of the patient are discussed further in Section 17.4 and are compared with the death certificate study and the prospective study.

7. Alleviation of pain and symptoms

7.1 Introduction

This chapter presents the results for questions related to the alleviation of pain and symptoms. The introduction to this series of questions was as follows:

I should like to ask a separate question about the alleviation of pain and symptoms. It happens from time to time that, in serious cases, pain and other symptoms can only be treated with high doses of morphine or morphine-like drugs. This can also shorten life.

In by far most of the cases the alleviation of pain and symptoms is the prime purpose of administering morphine or morphine-like drugs. Even though this is not the purpose these drugs can shorten life, but do not necessarily do so. If the pain suffered by a patient can be treated adequately, this can even act as life-prolonging, certainly with the dosage forms now available. As such, the use of these drugs is part of normal medical practice. If, however, morphine or morphine-like drugs are given with the express purpose of terminating life, this becomes euthanasia (provided this happens on request of the patient). These cases were discussed under this heading in Chapter 5. Nevertheless, it will become clear that there is a wide borderline area between these two situations.

7.2 Number of cases

The first question of this part of the questionnaire was: *"Did you ever face a situation in which you had to give such high doses of morphine or morphine-like drugs that it almost certainly would shorten the life of the patient?"* Table

Table 7.1   **The administration of doses of morphine or morphine-like drugs such that the patient's life was almost certainly shortened (physician interviews)**

	General practitioner n=152 %	Specialist n=202 %	Nursing home physician n=50 %	Total n=404 %
Administered at some time	82	81	86	82
Administered during the past year (one or more times)	52	66	78	58
Administration is conceivable	13	10	7	12
Would never do so	5	9	7	7
Total	100	100	100	100

7.1 provides information about the use of morphine or morphine-like drugs in such doses. All data in this chapter refer to this use of morphine and do not deal with all the situations in which morphine was used with no chance of shortening life.

More than 80% of respondents, regardless of specialty, indicated that they had at some time acted as described above. This had happened less than one year ago for more than half of the respondents.

With weighting for the total population of physicians in The Netherlands one can calculate from the answers to the above question that this happens annually in 16.3% of all deaths (95% confidence interval 15.3% to 17.4%). The treating physician is the general practitioner in about one third of the cases, the specialist in about half and the nursing home physician in the remaining cases.

7.3 Characteristics of the decision

It was stated in the introduction to this chapter that the concept of alleviation of pain and/or symptoms covers a wide variety of procedures. These differences are now illustrated using the most recent cases described by the respondents.

The differences in actions become clear when the intent of the physician is considered (Table 7.2). In most cases the physician intended to alleviate pain or other symptoms while it was taken into account that the life of the patient could be shortened. This probability then was "accepted". Thus, in about 65% of cases morphine was not used because of its possible life-shortening effect. In 30% of all cases termination of life was part of the physician's intent. In 6% it was the explicit purpose. In all these cases the patient had at some time indicated something about terminating life and an explicit request had been made in two thirds of the cases. This situation is therefore rather similar to euthanasia. The patient's wish is discussed further in Section 7.5. Shortening of life never had been the explicit purpose in the cases described by nursing home physicians.

A second differentiating characteristic was the supposed extent of shortening of life due to administration of morphine or morphine-like drugs. Table 7.3 shows the extent of life shortening. Life was shortened by maximally one week in about 70% of cases. Thus, this agrees with the extent of life shortening described in the previous chapter. Furthermore, according to the respondents, life was not shortened in about 8% of cases in spite of the use of morphine in high doses. Life was shortened by one to four weeks in a quarter of cases. The extent of shortening of life in general was much less than with euthanasia or assisted suicide.

Administering morphine or morphine-like drugs at doses that almost certainly shorten life differs in two other aspects from the situations described in Chapter 5. These aspects concern consultations with colleagues and filling in of the certificate of death.

Table 7.2 The intent of the physician when administering morphine in doses such that the patient's life was almost certainly shortened (physician interviews)

	General practitioner n=113 %	Specialist n=144 %	Nursing home physician n=40 %	Total n=297 %
Taking into account the probability that life would be shortened	66	59	78	65
Partly with the purpose of shortening life	29	33	23	30
With the explicit purpose of shortening life	5	8	–	6
Total	100	100	100	100

Table 7.3 Extent of shortening of life due to morphine administration in doses that almost certainly shortened life (physician interviews)

	General practitioner n=115 %	Specialist n=144 %	Nursing home physician n=39 %	Total n=298 %
No shortening	9	8	5	8
Less than 24 hours[1]		20	21	63
Up to one week	64	40	44	
1 to 4 weeks	26	28	18	26
1 to 6 months	2	4	13	3
More than half a year	–	0	–	0
Total	100	100	100	100

1) General practitioners only had 'up to one week' as a possible answer. No difference was thus made in their cases between 'less than 24 hours' and 'up to one week'.

Table 7.4 Consultations with colleagues, nursing staff and relatives when administering morphine in doses that almost certainly shortened life (physician interviews)

	General practitioner n=114 %	Specialist n=143 %	Nursing home physician n=41 %	Total n=298 %
Consultation with colleagues	38	71	41	47
Nursing staff involved with patient	80	100	100	87
Consultation with nursing staff (if involved with patient)	46	98	*100*	66
Consultation with relatives	64	72	60	66

Respondents occasionally consult colleagues, nursing staff and next of kin about administering morphine in high doses (Table 7.4). The percentages differ between types of physician. It is clear that one feels less need for a consultation about administering morphine (in high doses) than when a decision to perform euthanasia or assisted suicide is involved. This also is the reason most often stated (81%).

One can also consider the manner in which the death certificate was filled in. 'Natural death' was stated in all cases. In more than 90% of cases this happened because, in the opinion of the physician this was indeed a natural death. In about 9% of the cases this was done because it was felt that it would be troublesome to report an unnatural death.

7.4 Characteristics of the patient

Table 7.5 presents the distribution according to age and sex. The table also summarises the age and sex distribution of deaths in The Netherlands during 1990. The age distribution differs from that of the general population of The Netherlands in that these patients are, on the average, younger. The age distribution of the patient group was almost identical to that found for the group of patients where life was terminated without explicit request. Patients for whom euthanasia or assisted suicide was performed were, on the average, still younger.

Table 7.6 presents a summary of the most important diseases of the patients discussed above. The high incidence of cancer in this group of patients is noteworthy, as it was in the patients discussed in Chapters 5 and 6. Here also this

Table 7.5   Age and sex of patients receiving morphine in doses that almost certainly shortened life, compared to all deaths in the general population in The Netherlands (physician interviews)

Age	Deaths in the study		Deaths in the general population in the Netherlands in 1990[1]	
	Males n=175 %	Females n=125 %	Males n=66606 %	Females n=62180 %
	60	40	52	48
0 – 49	11	11	10	6
50 – 64	28	25	17	10
65 – 79	45	31	43	31
80+	17	33	31	53
Total	100	100	100	100

1)   Source: CBS causes-of-death statistics.

Table 7.6   Most important diseases of patients receiving morphine in doses that almost certainly shortened life (physician interviews)

	n=300 %	Distribution of causes of deaths in the general population in The Netherlands in 1990[1] n=128786 %
Cancer	77	27
Cardiovascular diseases	8	30
Diseases of the nervous system (incl. stroke)	5	12
Pulmonary diseases	3	8
Mental disorders	2	1
Others (all other categories)	6	22
Total	100	100

1)   Source: CBS causes-of-death statistics.

Table 7.7   Discussion with the patient when administering morphine in doses that almost certainly shortened life (physician interviews)

	General practitioner n=114 %	Specialist n=143 %	Nursing home physician n=41 %	Total n=298 %
Decision discussed with patient	40	41	29	39
Decision not discussed, patient totally able to take a decision	33	17	2	27
Decision not discussed, patient not (totally) able to take a decision	27	42	68	34
Total	100	100	100	100

percentage is much higher than that for the distribution of deaths in the general population (77% and 27% respectively).

7.5 Discussion with, and the wishes of the patient

Table 7.7 presents the percentage of cases in which the use of possibly life-shortening doses of morphine had been discussed with the patient, as different from the purpose for which this drug was used. In 39% of cases the administration of morphine in such doses had been discussed with the patient. In more than half of the patients where this discussion had not taken place the reason was inability of the patient to assess the situation and take a decision adequately.

Table 7.8   Degree of ability of patients to take a decision concerning administration of morphine in doses that almost certainly shortened life (physician interviews)

	General practitioner n=115 %	Specialist n=143 %	Nursing home physician n=41 %	Total n=299 %
Was the patient able to assess the situation and take a decision adequately?				
– totally able	71	54	27	63
– not totally able	13	17	10	13
– totally unable	17	29	64	23
Total	100	100	100	100
Most important cause of not being (totally) able)				
– *reduced consciousness*	*61*	*57*	*33*	*55*
– *demented*	*15*	*9*	*57*	*19*

1)   More than one answer could be given to this question.

Table 7.9   Previous wishes of patients with respect to terminating life (physician interviews)

	General practitioner n=115 %	Specialist n=143 %	Nursing home physician n=41 %	Total n=299 %
Patient had never indicated anything about terminating life	57	63	61	59
Patient had indicated at some time something about terminating life, but there was no explicit request	10	7	8	9
Patient had indicated at some time something about terminating life; the request was not strongly explicit	19	12	17	17
Patient had indicated at some time something; there was a strongly explicit request	15	18	14	15
Total	100	100	100	100

On the whole about one third of the patients were not (totally) able to assess the situation and take a decision adequately (Table 7.8). As could be expected, this percentage was considerably higher for nursing home physicians. The most important cause of inadequacy in patients treated by general practitioners and specialists was decreased consciousness, and dementia in patients of nursing home physicians.

Because life can be shortened by using morphine or morphine-like drugs (only at what are high doses for the patient), such drugs can also be used for this purpose. Therefore a question as to whether the patient had perhaps suggested something in this direction had been included in the questionnaire. The replies to this question are shown in Table 7.9.

As far as known to the physician, the patient had never indicated anything about termination of life in 59% of the cases; 40% of these patients were not (totally) able to take a decision. However, the patient very definitely had hinted at termination of life in 41% of cases. This varied from "I don't feel the need to carry on" or "I do not want you to prolong my life needlessly" to " I feel so much pain, please give me an injection". As already mentioned in Section 7.3, all cases for which the physician indicates that he had given morphine with the explicit purpose to shorten life are numbered among these 41%. There even was an explicit request of the patient to terminate life in 15% of the cases.

8. Non-treatment decisions

8.1 Introduction

This chapter deals with the replies to the questions about non-treatment decisions. First, the situation is discussed in which withdrawing treatment or withholding treatment happens on explicit request of the patient (Section 8.2). Thereafter cases are discussed in which treatment was withdrawn or withheld without explicit request of the patient (Section 8.3). The decision not to resuscitate is discussed in Section 8.4.

These three types of decisions appear to be so closely linked to the usual medical decision-making process that several respondents were not able to recall a concrete example, while they knew with certainty that they had taken this type of decision regularly. Moreover, the interviewers had been instructed that, should they be short of time, they should skip the questions discussed in Sections 8.2 and 8.3. This modification was necessary in about 20 interviews.

8.2 Non-treatment decisions upon the patient's request

8.2.1 Number of cases

The introduction to this series of cases was:

It happens in medical practice that a physician proposes some treatment but the patient prefers not to accept this. Even if a clearly life-prolonging treatment is under discussion the patient may prefer not to give permission to start this treatment. It can also happen that a patient explicitly requests that the current treatment be stopped, even if this treatment would clearly prolong life.

The respondent was first asked if he ever had experienced such a situation and if he had agreed to such a request by a patient. Of the physicians questioned, 71% answered in the affirmative.

To prevent each request by a patient, including all those requests that had definitely not contributed to a shortening of life, from being discussed in this part of the interview, the following limitation was added:

Have there also been situations in which a patient had asked explicitly that life-prolonging treatment not be started or be ceased, with at least in part the aim to shorten life?

In these cases the patient tried to shorten life by withdrawing or witholding

Table 8.1 Respondents who at some time withdrew or withheld a treatment upon request of the patient (physician interviews)

	General practitioner n=146 %	Specialist n=192 %	Nursing home physician n=50 %	Total n=388 %
Ever received and acted upon a request	65	83	76	71
Ever received and acted upon a request with (in part) the purpose of shortening life	45	47	53	46
Received one or more requests by a patient with (in part) the purpose of shortening life within the past 12 months	31	33	39	32

Tabel 8.2 Age and sex of patients in whom a treatment was withdrawn or withheld upon their request (physician interviews)

Age	Males n=91 %	Females n=78 %
	52	48
0-49	5	18
50-64	28	19
65-79	45	29
80+	23	34
Total	100	100

Table 8.3 Most important diseases of patients in whom a treatment was withdrawn or withheld upon their request (physician interviews)

	n=169 %
Cancer	64
Cardiovascular diseases	10
Diseases of the nervous system (incl. stroke)	9
Pulmonary diseases	2
Mental disorders	1
Others (all other categories)	14
Total	100

treatment. In this situation the intention of the patient is central and the physician may not agree with this intention. Obviously, decisions with respect to termination of life have been taken in consultation between physician and patient, but the physician did not necessarily have to agree to that decision. If a patient had withdrawn treatment, e.g. a medication, without consulting the physician, the case was not included in the description.

Requests by a patient that treatment be withdrawn or withheld with the intent to shorten life were experienced by 46% of the physicians. In the past year this had happened at least once to 32% of the respondents.

Based on the numbers supplied by the respondents one can estimate that, in The Netherlands, physicians receive some 5800 times annually the request to withdraw or withhold treatment with at least in part the intent to shorten life. About 3300 of these requests are directed to the general practitioner, about 600 to the nursing home physician and the remainder the specialist.

8.2.2 Characteristics of the patient

Following the questions as to the frequency of this type of decision, detailed questions were asked about the most recent case of this type. The distribution of age and sex are shown in Table 8.2. Comparison to the general population in The Netherlands was omitted because not all patients had died at the time the interview took place. In total, 18% of the patients discussed here were alive at the time of the interview.

The most important diseases of the patients discussed in this part of the interview are shown in Table 8.3. The high incidence of cancer is again noticeable (64%).

8.2.3 The request of the patient

As was the case in Chapter 5, the request of the patient plays a crucial role in the decisions discussed here, whether withold or withdraw a treatment. Table 8.4 shows that in the majority of cases an explicit and strong request was involved. In the opinion of the respondents, the request almost always originated completely from the patients themselves. The respondent felt that, in almost all cases, the patient was able to assess his situation at the time the request was made and could take the decision adequately.

The most frequent reason for the patient to make the request was, according to respondents, the burden caused by the treatment. Other reasons mentioned often were loss of dignity, tiredness of life (particularly by nursing home patients) and the feeling of dependence.

The respondents mentioned pain in 22% of cases. In one case pain was the only reason; tiredness of life was mentioned as the only reason by 13 patients.

Table 8.4   **The request of the patient to withdraw or withhold a treatment (physician interviews)**

	General practitioner n=62 %	Specialist n=80 %	Nursing home physician n=27 %	Total n=169 %
Request strong and explicit	87	89	96	89
Written advance directive present	11	4	7	9
Request made completely by the patient himself	95	97	100	96
Patient totally able to take a decision	95	97	93	95
Most frequent reason for the patient's request[1]):				
– burden of treatment	45	46	16	43
– loss of dignity	27	32	52	31
– tiredness of life	23	31	68	28
– dependence	19	30	36	24

1)   More than one answer could be given to this question.

Table 8.5   **Consultation with others than the patient concerning the decision to withdraw or withhold a treatment[1]) (physician interviews)**

	General practitioner n=62 %	Specialist n=78 %	Nursing home physician n=26 %	Total n=166 %
Consultation with colleagues	31	67	65	43
Consultation with nursing staff	13	35	85	25
Consultation with relatives	42	42	65	44
Consultation with pastor or spiritual adviser	5	3	12	5
No one consulted	31	22	8	26

1)   More than one answer could be given to this question.

Table 8.6   **Extent of shortening of life due to withdrawing or withholding a treatment upon request of the patient[1]) (physician interviews)**

	General practitioner n=45 %	Specialist n=61 %	Nursing home physician n=23 %	Total n=129 %
No shortening	24	10	9	19
Less than 24 hours[2])	–	–	–	–
Up to one week	22	10	17	18
1 to 4 weeks	18	11	13	16
1 to 6 months	29	49	26	34
More than half a year	7	21	35	13
Total	100	100	100	100

1)   This question was only asked if the patient had died in the meanwhile. This was the case in 82% of patients.

2)   General practitioners only had 'up to one week' as a possible answer. No difference was thus made in their cases between 'less than 24 hours' and 'up to one week'.

8.2.4 Characteristics of the decision

Even if, in a great many cases (75%), the wish of the patient was the most important reason for the physician to accede to the patient's request, this does not complete the process of decision making. Specialists and nursing home physicians had consultations concerning their decision in two thirds of the cases, and general practitioners in one third of cases. Nursing staff was consulted in about one quarter of cases (Table 8.5). In these cases it is not known in how many instances there were no nursing staff, partner or other relatives members available.

If the patient had died in the meanwhile respondents were asked for their estimate of by how much the patient's life was shortened due to withdrawing or withholding treatment. The results are shown in Table 8.6.

A remarkable picture emerges on comparison of the estimated extent of shortening life with that due to euthanasia and assisted suicide (see Table 5.13). Particularly in the case of the specialists, shortening of life due to euthanasia and assisted suicide was less than the shortening due to withdrawing or withholding treatment upon request of the patient, (in part) with the purpose of shortening life.

As was the case in Chapter 7, that dealt with alleviation of pain and symptoms, the question was asked here as to the intent of the decision to withdraw or withhold treatment. However, there are two important differences. In the situation discussed here everything is focussed on the patient's decision. Contrary to the situation in which the patient requests euthanasia or assisted suicide there is less room here for a role of the physician: the patient has the right to refuse treatment. The patient's intention does not have to agree with that of the physician.

Secondly, at the beginning of this series of questions the 'condition' was put that only cases should be discussed in which the patient (in part) intended to die. The category of chapter 7 'taking into account the probability that this decision would hasten the end of life' therefore is not one of the possible categories that were answered in table 8.7. This table shows that in about one quarter of cases shortening of life was an explicit aim. In the other cases this aim seems to have been less dominant in the physician's thinking.

In cases where the patient had died in the meanwhile it was asked how the death certificate had been filled in. In all but one case the physician had declared that a natural death was involved. This single case was a patient who had had an accident with a spinal cord lesion ("broken neck") who had asked specifically to have the respirator switched off. Considering that the accident was the cause of death, no declaration of a natural death was made.

It should not be surprising that, in several cases, treatment was withdrawn or

Table 8.7   Intention behind the decision to withdraw or withhold a treatment (physician interviews)

	General practitioner n=52 %	Specialist n=59 %	Nursing home physician n=23 %	Total n=134 %
Partly with the purpose of shortening life	83	56	57	74
With the explicit purpose of shortening life	17	44	44	26
Total	100	100	100	100

withheld with the explicit purpose of shortening life while a declaration of natural death was made. Death is considered natural as long as it was upon request of the patient that treatment was withheld (see draft of law on euthanasia from 1987). Nevertheless several respondents (7% of general practitioners and 2% of specialists) indicated that they had not reported an unnatural death because reporting was troublesome.

8.3 Non-treatment decisions without explicit request of the patient

8.3.1 Number of cases

Cases were discussed in the first part of this chapter in which treatment was withdrawn or withheld upon explicit request of the patient. The discontinuation of a treatment without an explicit request of the patient is discussed here.

The introduction in the questionnaire was as follows:

The decision to withhold or to withdraw a current treatment * *or not to perform certain types of diagnostic procedures are daily decisions in medical practice. In most instances this concerns situations in which the treating physician does not expect or does not observe sufficient success. However, there are situations in which a considerable life-prolonging effect can be expected from a certain treatment while the decision can nevertheless be made to withhold such*

---

*   In this investigation, tube feed is also considered as treatment.

treatment or to withdraw it. This implies that under such circumstances considerable prolongation of life is considered undesirable or even futile. 'Considerable' is taken to mean more than one month.

We have already discussed situations in which a patient requests that treatment be withheld or withdrawn. I should now like to discuss with you situations in which such a decision is taken without the request or without the explicit request of the patient.

Briefly, two types of situations are discussed here. On the one hand therapies are involved which will probably meet with little or no success. Such treatment can be withdrawn or withheld for this reason. On the other hand there are cases in which therapies which can have a considerable (more than one month) life-prolonging effect but in which prolongation of life is undesirable or pointless and treatment is withdrawn or withheld for this reason.

It was intended to discuss only the second type of decision situation. This was aimed at preventing mainly the day-to-day decisions by the physician to treat or not to treat from being discussed, with shortening of life probably playing no role whatsoever. It was expected that when discussing the second type of decision the emphasis would shift toward possibly more 'weighty' decisions. It seemed from the case descriptions and the replies to the question as to the extent of shortening of life, that both types of decision were nevertheless described.

It should be mentioned that several respondents described patients meeting criteria for cerebral death. These cases were not included in the description because in such cases there is no question of a medical decision with death as (possible) consequence but of withdrawing treatment because the patient already is 'dead'. However, one could also conclude from these responses that some physicians consider withdrawing treatment of a brain-dead patient as an important decision.

The first question asked was whether the physician had ever decided to withhold a life-prolonging treatment or to withdraw one, without the explicit request of the patient. Table 8.8 shows that almost two thirds of the physicians indicated that they have taken such a decision at some time. All but one of the nursing home physicians have taken such a decision at some time. This figure is about one half for general practitioners. Half of the physicians had taken such a decision at least once during the past year. There is a clear difference between general practitioners, specialists and nursing home physicians (38%, 68% and 96% respectively) here also.

Only a small fraction of the physicians, 14%, would never withdraw or withhold treatment without explicit request of the patient. All nursing home physicians see this type of situation as conceivable.

Based on the numbers obtained one can estimate that in The Netherlands such a decision is taken 25 000 times annually. The general practitioner takes the

Table 8.8   Respondents who withdrew or withheld a life-prolonging treatment at some time without explicit request of the patient (physician interviews)

	General practitioner n=144 %	Specialist n=190 %	Nursing home physician n=50 %	Total n=384 %
Treatment withdrawn or withheld at some time without explicit request of patient	51	80	98	62
Treatment withdrawn or withheld without explicit request of the patient within the past 12 monthst	38	68	96	50
Is conceivable	32	10	2	24
Would never withdraw or withhold treatment without explicit request of patient	17	9	–	14
Total	100	100	100	100

decision in 6000 cases, the nursing home physician does so in 5000 and the specialist in 14 000 cases.

8.3.2 Characteristics of the patient

In the interview questions were asked about the last time a treatment was withdrawn or withheld without explicit request of the patient. The patient

Table 8.9   Age and sex of patients for whom a treatment was withdrawn or withheld without explicit request (physician interview)

Age	Males n=114 %	Females n=146 %
	37	63
0-49	12	5
50-64	14	7
65-79	37	27
80+	37	62
Total	100	100

involved need not have died. The percentages in the tables refer to the most recent case.

With respect to age and sex distribution it is noteworthy that withdrawing treatment or withholding treatment without explicit request of the patient occurs much more often with women than with men (see Table 8.9). One of the explanations is that relatively older patients are involved.

Table 8.10 shows the distribution over the most important disease groups. In the situations discussed in the previous chapters cancer always occurred relatively frequently as compared to the total distribution of causes of death. In the situation discussed here, one third of the patients suffered from cancer, 14% from a cardiovascular disease, 14% from a disease of the central nervous system and 17% from pulmonary disease. Thus the decision discussed in this section is much more regularly distributed over disease groups. This is consistent with the fact that generally older patients are involved. Although the absolute number of patients dying from cancer is highest in the oldest age group (80+), the relative incidence of cancer in the total number of deaths is considerably less than in the younger age groups.

8.3.3 The request of the patient

The decisions discussed here were taken without explicit request of the patient. This does not imply that patients may not have made some reference to terminating life in some cases. An implicit question was often involved about no longer prolonging life should this not be reasonable. In total, 18% of patients had indicated something in this manner, as is shown in table 8.11 but only 1% actually recorded this in a written advance directive. The decision not to treat was discussed in 13% of all cases.

In 79% of the cases (see Table 8.12) when the physician had taken the decision not to treat he considered the patient not totally able or unable to assess the situation and take a decision adequately at the time. This was reason for the physicians not to discuss this decision with the patient. The cause for this lack of ability of the patient to take a decision was primarily loss of consciousness or dementia.

8.3.4 Characteristics of the decision

Although in most cases the physician did not discuss it with the patient, he did consult others in almost all instances. The physician consulted a colleague in more than half the cases. Nursing staff and relatives were consulted in more than half the cases (Table 8.13). It is not known in how many instances no nursing staff, partner or other relatives were available.

Table 8.10 **Most important diseases of patients for whom a treatment was withdrawn or withheld without their explicit request (physician interviews)**

	n=260 %
Cancer	35
Cardiovascular diseases	14
Diseases of the nervous system (incl. stroke)	14
Pulmonary diseases	17
Mental disorders	3
Others (all other categories)	17
Totaal	100

Table 8.11 **Earlier wishes by and discussion with patients for whom a treatment was withdrawn or withheld without their explicit request (physician interviews)**

	General practitioner n=70 %	Specialist n=142 %	Nursing home physician n=48 %	Total n=260 %
Patient indicated something at some time about terminating life	21	13	21	18
Decision discussed with patient	10	20	6	13
Written advance directive available	–	1	2	1

Table 8.12 **Degree of ability to take a decision of patients for whom a treatment was withdrawn or withheld (physician interviews)**

	General practitioner n=70 %	Specialist n=142 %	Nursing home physician n=48 %	Total n=260 %
Patient able to assess the situation and take a decision adequately?				
– totally able	21	26	8	22
– not totally able	27	14	10	21
– unable	51	60	81	58
Total	100	100	100	100
Most important cause for being not (totally) able [1]				
– *temporarily unconscious*	*6*	*8*	*2*	*6*
– *permanently unconscious*	*7*	*33*	*9*	*16*
– *reduced consciousness*	*39*	*37*	*34*	*38*
– *demented*	*41*	*25*	*68*	*39*

1) More than one answer could be given to this question.

Table 8.13 Consultation with others than the patient concerning the decision to withdraw or withhold a treatment without explicit request of the patient[1] (physician interviews)

	General practitioner n=70 %	Specialist n=142 %	Nursing home physician n=48 %	Total n=260 %
Consultation with colleagues	33	86	56	54
Consultation with nursing staff	49	56	94	56
Consultation with relatives	63	49	81	60
Consultation with pastor or spiritual adviser	1	2	10	3
No consultation	10	6	2	8

1) More than one answer could be given to this question.

Table 8.14 shows the extent of shortening of life in those cases in which the patient died. In 56% of the cases life was shortened by up to one week by withdrawing treatment. Life was shortened by more than half a year in 7% of cases. This table also shows that the introduction to this series of questions which restricted the selection to cases with shortening of life by more than one month was interpreted rather broadly by the respondents.

As described for the cases in Chapter 7, the question was also asked here as to the intention of the physician in deciding to withhold or withdraw treatment. In two thirds of the cases the physicians took into account the probability that the life of the patient would be shortened. However, in 16% of cases shortening of life was the explicit purpose. Table 8.15 presents the intentions of the physicians.

The death certificate almost always stated 'natural death' because, in the opinion of the physicians, this almost always had been the case. According to the physicians only in four cases it had not been a natural death. Three of these were not reported as such. One case was reported because it concerned a (not completely successful) suicide.

8.4 'Do not resuscitate' decisions

8.4.1 Number of decisions not to resuscitate

Sections 8.2 and 8.3 included discussions about withholding treatment. These cases were concerned with an actual choice between starting a treatment at that moment or not doing so. This section deals with anticipatory decisions. This implies that a decision is taken regarding a situation that might arise in the future. An agreement not to resuscitate belongs to this type of decision. This type of decision is part of the category MDELs because a decision is taken that (possibly) will shorten the life of the patient. However, a decision not to resuscitate can be seen somewhat as an exception because in most cases it does

Table 8.14 **Extent of shortening of life due to withdrawing or withholding a treatment without explicit request of the patient[1]) (physician interviews)**

	General practitioner n=60 %	Specialist n=112 %	Nursing home physician n=41 %	Total n=213 %
No shortening	22	18	15	20
Less than 24 hours[2])		13	5	36
Up to one week	38	25	20	
1 to 4 weeks	20	26	22	22
1 to 6 months	13	12	32	15
More than half a year	7	7	7	7
Total	100	100	100	100

1) This question was asked only if the patient had died in the meanwhile. This was the case in 90% of cases.

2) General practitioners only had 'up to one week' as a possible answer. No difference was thus made in their cases between 'less than 24 hours' and 'up to one week'.

Table 8.15 **Intentions of physicians who withdrew or withheld a treatment without explicit request of the patient (physician interviews)**

	General practitioner n=66 %	Specialist n=137 %	Nursing home physician n=45 %	Total n=248 %
Taking into account the probability that life would be shortened	64	66	71	65
Partly with the purpose to shorten life	21	15	18	19
With the explicit purpose to shorten life	15	20	11	16
Total	100	100	100	100

not need to be carried out: the decision is thus not followed by action.

Although the precise description of the term 'resuscitate' will depend on the facilities the physician has available, it can be assumed that in any case all physicians will include heart massage and some form of artificial respiration (basic life support).

The introduction to the series of question was as follows:

There are situations in which it is agreed explicitly that a patient will not be resuscitated if (functional) cardiac or respiratory arrest occurs. This anticipating decision is named a DNR or NTBR * decision. The initiative for such a decision is usually taken by the physician, but sometimes by the patient. Thus, this situation differs from the one that arises only once arrest has occurred.

Table 8.16 shows that it is particularly specialists who frequently take decisions not to resuscitate. All specialists who were interviewed had taken a decision not to resuscitate at some time and in almost all cases this had happened once or more during the past year. The figures for nursing home physicians are quite different. The reason appears to be that there is the implicit agreement, in many nursing homes, not to resuscitate in principle. The reply of 40% of the nursing home physicians was that they had never explicitly taken the decision not to resuscitate.

Extrapolating to annual figures one can calculate that some 91 000 decisions not to resuscitate are taken in hospitals each year. This amounts to approximately 6% of all admissions to hospital. The existence of the decision not to resuscitate certainly does not imply that a patient will die during admission (Chapter 17). Nursing home physicians take decisions not to resuscitate 3100 times annually, general practitioners do so 3000 times.

These answers show that there are distinct differences between general practioners on the one hand and specialists and nursing home physicians on the

Table 8.16 **Respondents who at some time have taken a decision not to resuscitate (physician interviews)**

	General practitioner n=143 %	Specialist total n=200 %	Nursing home physician n=50 %
DNR decision taken at some time	21	100	40
Taken a DNR decision one or more times during the past year	15	96	33
Never taken a DNR decision, but decision conceivable	69	–	18
DNR decision inconceivable because I refuse to do this	6	–	2
DNR decision inconceivable because resuscitation is never carried out in the institution / I do not do this	4	–	40
Total	100	100	100

*   DNR: 'do not resuscitate', NTBR: 'not to be resuscitated'

Table 8.17   **Most important diseases of patients for whom a DNR decision was taken (physician interviews)**

	n=203 %
Cancer	35
Cardiovascular diseases	22
Diseases of the nervous system (incl. stroke)	16
Pulmonary diseases	9
Mental disorders	3
Others (all other categories)	16
Total	100

other. Only 30 (21%) of 143 general practitioners who answered this question ever took a decision not to resuscitate. Ten of these physicians had taken the decision more than a year ago.

The data on general practitioners are not presented because decisions not to resuscitate occur relatively infrequently among these physicians. The remaining tables of this section present only data for specialists and nursing home physicians. Furthermore, it is of interest that general practitioners relatively often take the decision not to resuscitate at the moment the patient requests not to receive any further treatment. This situation occurred in almost half of the DNR decisions by general practitioners. This observation also suggests that general practitioners arrive at such decisions differently from the other types of physicians discussed here.

8.4.2 Characteristics of patients and the decision-making process

The most important diseases of patients for whom DNR decisions were taken by specialists and nursing home physicians are presented in Table 8.17.

The respondents were also asked if the decision not to resuscitate had been discussed with the patient, whether the patient was able to assess the situation and take a decision adequately. The specialists had discussed the DNR decision with the patient in 14% of cases, the nursing home physicians had done so in 28%. Specialists did not discuss this decision with the patient in 30% of cases in which the patient was able to assess the situation and take a decision adequately. For the nursing home physicians this amounted to 17% of the cases.

There seldom were written advance directives for the specialists' patients (4%), and there were none for nursing home patients. These figures represent the total of resuscitation and other written advance directives concerning the termination of life.

Finally respondents were questioned about their most important considerations when taking a DNR decision and about possible consultation with others than the patient. The most important reasons for the specialists not to resuscitate were: the prognosis of the disease (mentioned in 57% of cases), no chance for improvement (54%), poor quality of life of the patient (28%), resuscitation would have had no chance of success (27%) and the wishes of the patient (8%). Nursing home physicians gave the same reasons as the specialists but mentioned the poor quality of life and the wishes of the patient more frequently.

Specialists consulted colleagues concerning DNR decisions in three quarters of cases and nursing staff in nearly the same number of cases.

9. Physicians' opinions

9.1 Introduction

Respondents were asked several questions about their knowledge concerning the rules of due care with respect to euthanasia and about their views on euthanasia. When respondents' views were discussed, the issues covered included their opinion about the rules of due care with respect to euthanasia, the reporting or not reporting of an unnatural death, the role of the nursing staff when decisions were being taken and the opinion of the respondent with respect to proposals for laws.

A remark should be made here about the significance of the data presented. The sample was structured so that representative information could be gathered for most of the deaths (see Chapter 4). This aim could be achieved in a study based on interviews with general practitioners, nursing home physicians and five types of specialists. Specialties with relatively few deaths were therefore not considered while obviously, members of such specialties also have opinions. The distribution of opinions as presented in this chapter does not hold for all physicians in The Netherlands but does hold for almost all types of physicians who deal with dying patients regularly. This limitation is of particular importance for specialists working in hospital.

9.2 Rules of due care with respect to euthanasia

Almost all physicians answered in the affirmative the question "Are you aware of the existence of the rules of due care with respect to euthanasia?" (Table 9.1).

The respondent was then asked to mention several rules of due care. Table 9.1 summarises both the rules of due care as formulated by the KNMG, the Health Council or in the 1987 proposal of law, and the percentage of respondents that mentioned one or more of these rules spontaneously. Respondents mentioned an average of 3.3 rules of due care. Almost all respondents who were aware of the existence of rules of due care mentioned consultation with colleagues, about two thirds mentioned the seriously considered request of the patients; all other rules were mentioned less frequently. Of the physicians involved, 76% mentioned at least one of the three rules concerning the request of the patient ('free will', 'seriously considered request', 'long-standing desire'). The fact that free choice was mentioned by fewer than half the respondents however, does not necessarily mean that this would not be a grave consideration for the other respondents. It could simply have been considered as obvious.

The fact that voluntariness regarding the request (for euthanasia) was considered obvious is confirmed by the data of Table 9.2. Respondents were

Table 9.1   **Respondents' knowledge of the rules of due care with respect to euthanasia (physician interviews)**

	General practitioner n=152 %	Specialist n=202 %	Nursing home physician n=50 %	Total n=404 %
Aware of the existence of rules of due care	99	94	100	98
If above question is answered affirmatively:				
Rules of due care mentioned ¹):				
− *voluntariness*	*42*	*40*	*49*	*42*
− *seriously considered request*	*71*	*54*	*76*	*66*
− *long-standing desire to die*	*16*	*15*	*47*	*18*
− *suffering not acceptable for patient*	*41*	*26*	*37*	*37*
− *consultation with colleague*	*90*	*87*	*94*	*89*
− *explanation of diagnosis, course of illness and alternative therapies*	*10*	*13*	*18*	*11*
− *relatives were informed unless patient did not wish this*	*15*	*23*	*2*	*16*
− *written report on decision-taking*	*44*	*23*	*25*	*37*

1)   More than one reply could be given to this question.

Table 9.2   **Opinion regarding rules of due care; percentages of physicians who consider the rule stated (very) important (physician interviews)**

	General practitioner n=151 %	Specialist n=201 %	Nursing home physician n=50 %	Total n=402 %
Voluntariness	98	97	98	98
Seriously considered request	99	97	100	99
Long-standing desire to die	75	69	90	74
Unacceptable suffering for patient	95	94	96	95
Consultation with colleague	60	79	90	67
Information about diagnosis, course of the illness and treatment alternatives	90	98	94	93
Relatives were informed unless patient did not wish this	72	73	80	73
Written report	51	70	92	59
No treatment alternatives	57	78	74	64
Technically faultless performance	99	97	100	99
Incurable disease	78	89	66	81
Patient dying	66	59	40	63
Nursing staff must be involved in making decision	33	73	82	47
No unnecessary suffering for others	40	57	52	46

asked to indicate their view of the degree of importance of several official and unofficial rules of due care on a scale from 1 to 5. Most respondents felt that free choice, the carefully considered request and the technically faultless performance were particularly important or very important. Although all respondents mentioned consultation with colleagues as one of the rules of due care, not all respondents found this important or very important. Of the general practitioners, 40% did not feel that consultation is (very) important.

Almost an identical distribution was found for replies to the separate question *"Do you feel that a colleague should be consulted in all cases of euthanasia?"*: almost 40% of the general practitioners replied in the negative, as did 14% of specialists and 10% of nursing home physicians, respectively.

9.3 Examining and reporting

About two thirds of specialists and nursing home physicians answered in the affirmative to the question *"Do you feel that each case of euthanasia should somehow examined?"* About 30% felt that this is sometimes but not always

Table 9.3   **Examination of euthanasia; opinions of specialists and nursing home physicians (physician interviews)**

	Specialist n=199 %		Nursing home physician n=50 %		Total n=249 %	
Do you feel that each case of euthanasia should somehow be examined?						
– yes	61		76		64	
– no, but sometimes yes	31		22		29	
– no, never	9		2		7	
Total	100		100		100	
Only for respondents answering 'yes' or 'sometimes' to the above stated question:						
Who should test in 1st or 2nd instance (see text)[1]	1st	2nd	1st	2nd	1st	2nd
– Public prosecutor	7	25	25	49	10	30
– Medical tribunal	2	17	4	31	2	20
– Coroner	8	3	10	6	9	3
– Health inspector	15	38	14	35	15	37
– Medical-ethical committee	35	11	37	12	35	11
– Institutional committee of colleagues	52	11	27	2	47	9
– Independent medical examiner	30	16	35	6	31	14
– Other	12	10	8	4	12	9

1)   More than one answer could be given to this question.

necessary and a small minority felt that euthanasia need never be examined. It is not possible to determine whether all the respondents interpreted this question the same way. It could have been seen as referring only to legal examination (Table 9.3). Those who felt that all or only some cases of euthanasia needed to be examined were asked subsequently who should examine a case of euthanasia or assisted suicide in the first instance and who in second instance, in cases that could not pass the examination in the first instance. In the opinion of specialists and nursing home physicians, physicians are the candidates of choice for performing the first examination. A medical-ethical committee, an institutional committee of colleagues or an independent medical examiner would be suitable. If a case does not pass the first examination, a health inspector or public prosecutor could be considered for the next examination.

The question concerning the examining of euthanasia was put in a different manner to general practitioners, who had been interviewed on the basis of an earlier version of the questionnaire.

The question: *"Do you feel that each case of euthanasia should be examined legally?"* was answered in the affirmative by 30% of general practitioners. The following question: "Do you feel that in each case of euthanasia it would be sufficient to use in first instance a form of examination to be performed by colleagues according to a fixed protocol?" was answered in the affirmative by 69%. Some 15% of general practitioners added comments to their answers (e.g. "yes, legally but not by a criminal judge").

All respondents were also asked what would be the conditions under which they would be prepared to report truthfully that euthanasia had been performed. The question was put as follows: *"What would be the conditions under which you feel that one can require a physician to report to the police, coroner or legal authority a case of euthanasia as an unnatural death?"*

The answers are presented in Table 9.4. Respondents had to formulate the conditions themselves. No possible answers were offered.

More than a quarter of the physicians felt that euthanasia should always be reported as unnatural death; 22% of physicians felt that this could never be demanded from a physician. One out of three general practitioners mentions as condition that relatives must not be questioned by police. One quarter of physicians mentions prosecution as objection to reporting euthanasia.

In the proposals for a modified procedure (put forward by 20% of all respondents) emphasis was often placed on the fact that police must proceed with discretion. Many physicians who make this kind of suggestions emphasise that they would be prepared to report euthanasia as such but do not wish to be considered as suspect in a criminal act. Also the uncertainty of what might happen to the physician is considered as an obstacle to making a report of unnatural death. Physicians indicate that they need a careful, clearly formulated procedure that would not be drawn out for months on end.

Table 9.4 Under what conditions would physicians be prepared to report euthanasia as euthanasia to police, coroner or legal authority[1]) (physician interviews)

	General practitioner n=149 %	Specialist n=201 %	Nursing home physician n=49 %	Total n=399 %
Always	23	29	51	27
Only under the following conditions:				
– if reporting does not lead to questioning of relatives by police	35	20	22	30
– if reporting does not lead to prosecution	22	29	29	24
– if reporting procedure is modified, i.e. (see text)	21	18	14	20
– if reporting does not lead to confiscation of body	15	9	12	13
– if rules of due care were not applied	3	3	–	3
– if considerable life-shortening was involved	2	4	–	3
Under no condition	26	17	8	22
Other	7	8	4	7

1) More than one answer could be given to this question.

9.4 Role of nursing staff in euthanasia

It was not possible to interview a large number of nursing staff individually in the framework of this study (Chapter 2). However, a question about consulting nursing staff was asked for each MDEL. Moreover, several questions were asked about the role of nursing staff in euthanasia when questions about opinions were asked.

The first question as to the role of nursing staff referred to transmission to the physician of a request of the patient for euthanasia or assisted suicide. Respondents say that they had first heard from nursing staff about a patient's request for euthanasia or assisted suicide in 30% of cases.

This percentage differed somewhat for the different types of physicians: 15% of general practitioners, 60% of specialists and 50% of nursing home physicians.

It was asked next whether, in the respondent's experience, a nurse had ever taken the initiative to raise the topic of euthanasia with the physician without the patient's request. General practitioners had experienced this in 10% of cases, specialists and nursing home physicians in 31% and 26% of the cases, respectively.

Physicians were asked a question about the tasks of nursing staff in cases of euthanasia (see Table 9.5). Several possible replies were offered to the respondents. If necessary, the interviewer explained that 'task' had to be understood quite strictly. The issue thus arises of whether in the opinion of the physician the particular activity becomes an essential part of adequate functioning of the nurse.

The replies show that physicians consider in the first place that it is the task

Table 9.5   Opinion of physicians about the task of nursing staff in euthanasia (physician interviews)

	General practitioner n=150 %	Specialist n=200 %	Nursing home physician n=50 %	Total n=400 %
With reference to euthanasia, do you consider it the task of the nursing staff to: [1]				
– report the request of the patient	73	85	86	77
– introduce the topic	42	45	44	43
– look after the patient	61	66	68	63
– discuss the condition of the patient	91	76	82	86
– discuss the request of the patien	68	84	76	73
– discuss the intention of the physician	37	56	42	42
– be present when euthanasia is performed	11	26	22	16

[1]   More than one reply could be given to this question.

Table 9.6   Should nursing staff be permitted to perform euthanasia (physician interviews)

	General practitioner n=152 %	Specialist n=200 %	Nursing home physician n=50 %	Total n=402 %
Should a nurse be permitted to perform the act? [1]				
– never	94	72	92	88
– in my presence	2	18	2	7
– upon my request	2	14	4	6
– always	1	–	–	0
– other	2	6	2	3

[1] More than one answer could be given to this question.

of nursing staff to discuss with the physician the condition of and the request of the patient, to indicate that the patient has made a request and to look after the patient.

Respondents were also asked if nursing staff should be permitted to actually perform euthanasia. Here also, the respondents were offered possible answers. Almost all general practitioners and nursing home physicians felt that this should never be allowed; 72% of the specialists felt the same way (Table 9.6).

9.5 Other opinions

Twelve statements were presented to the physicians. Respondents were requested to indicate on a scale from 1 to 5 the extent to which they agreed with the particular statement. The 5 choices on the scale were:

— completely in agreement
— agree more than disagree
— neither agree nor disagree
— disagree more than agree
— completely in disagreement

Table 9.7 summarises the percentages of respondents that selected one of the first two choices (agreeing completely or partly).

Two thirds of the general practitioners feel that in certain situations it is up to the physician to raise the topic of euthanasia; this feeling is considerably less strong in the two other groups of physicians. Two thirds of the physicians feel that people have the right to decide over their own life and death. More than 90% of physicians feel that a physician must be able to count on not being prosecuted if all rules of due care have been met. This is in agreement with a finding from an earlier investigation [9]. Also, about 90% of physicians feel that euthanasia must only be performed by a physician. About 40% of physicians agree with the view voiced from time to time by opponents of euthanasia that adequate alleviation of pain and/or symptoms and appropriate care of the dying patient makes euthanasia unnecessary. Less than one third of the physicians believe that that the number of cases of euthanasia would increase if euthanasia were no longer punishable. Only a very small part of the respondents see a relationship between the incidence of requests for euthanasia and economic difficulties. Finally, more than three quarters of the physicians agree that euthanasia has become too much a politically charged topic.

9.6 Legislation

All respondents were asked a question concerning their wishes with respect to legislation covering euthanasia. The formulation of the question was:

Table 9.7   Opinions about some statements; percentages of physicians who (completely) agree (physician interviews)

	General practitioner n=152 %	Specialist n=202 %	Nursing home physician n=50 %	Total n=404 %
There can be situations in which the physician should raise euthanasia as a possibility with the patient	65	36	24	54
Everyone is entitled to decide over their own life and death	65	62	70	64
An institution should formulate its own policy regarding euthanasia	77	82	90	79
In spite of the possible existence of an institutional policy on euthanasia it is up to the psysician to decide wether or not to perform euthanasia	89	84	88	87
If under present-day circumstances all rules of due care have been met, a physician should be able to count on not being prosecuted	93	96	90	94
Euthanasia must only be performed by a physician	91	90	88	91
Adequate alleviation of pain and/or symptoms and personal care of the dying patient make euthanasia unnecessary	37	46	42	40
If patients know that a physician is prepared to perform euthanasia if really necessary they will request euthanasia less quickly	46	34	40	42
If euthanasia would no longer be punishable the number of cases of euthanasia would increase	29	37	26	31
In times of economic difficulties the number of requests for euthanasia will increase	9	8	6	8
The fuss now made about euthanasia is unnecessary, there always has been euthanasia	63	57	34	59
Euthanasia has become too much of a politically charged topic	77	83	74	79

1. *In the present situation euthanasia is, in principle, punishable but the public prosecutor will probably drop charges if it is clear that the physician has met several rules of due care. Here the principle is: "punishable unless".*

2. *Proposed legislation by the Second Chamber of Parliament (comparable to the House of Commons or House of Representatives) has as starting point that euthanasia is not punishable but that the physician's performance will be examined according to a procedure defined by law. Euthanasia is defined very strictly (by means of rules of due care). All acts leading to termination of life and falling outside this definition remain punishable. The principle here is: ''not punishable, provided''.*

3. *Finally there is proposed legislation from the previous cabinet in which euthanasia remains punishable in principle and the physician's acts will be examined by a procedure of law. At the same time the law determines the circumstances (rules of due care) that will absolve the physician. All acts leading to termination of life that fall outside these conditions remain punishable. The principle here is: ''punishable unless''.*

Do you have a preference for one of these situations?

Table 9.8 summarises the replies. A wrong card for the reply was offered to 41 specialists and their replies are thus not included in the tabulated data.

Two thirds of respondents prefer the draft law proposed by the Second Chamber described under 2. These results agree with the description of physicans' opinions about testing and reporting of euthanasia in Section 9.3: physicians do not wish to be considered as suspects and treated as suspected of

Table 9.8   **Opinions of physicians concerning legislation for euthanasia (physician interviews)**

	General practitioners n=152 %	Specialist n=160 %	Nursing home physician n=50 %	Total n=362 %
"Punishable unless" (situation 1)	7	12	2	8
"Not punishable provided" (situation 2)	67	64	62	66
"Punishable unless" but change of legislation in which "unless" is defined (situation 3)	11	11	22	12
Never punishable	7	6	2	7
Always punishable	1	–	–	1
Other	6	7	12	7
Total	100	100	100	100

having performed a criminal act after having acted along the rules of due care. A total of 15% of physicians indicate that they do not wish to choose from one of the three proposals shown above but they favour still another principle for legislation.

9.7 Philosophy of life

The question *"Do you consider yourself as belonging to a religious group or do you feel you adhere to a specific philosophy of life?"* was answered affirmatively by more than 40% of general practitioners and specialists and by 62% of nursing home physicians.

Most of those replying in the affirmative to this question indicate that this aspect plays a role in determining their point of view on euthanasia. This means that about one third of all physicians allow religion or philosophy of life to play a role with respect their attitude towards euthanasia, while 18% of physicians state that they consider this as very important (Table 9.9).

Table 9.9   Philosophy of life of respondents (physician interviews)

	General practitioners n=152 %	Specialist n=202 %	Nursing home physician n=50 %	Total n=404 %
Belonging to a religious group or linked to a specific philosophy of life	42	41	62	43
The above is important in determining the point of view regarding euthanasia:				
− not	12	14	18	13
− somewhat	10	13	20	12
− important	20	14	24	18
− not applicable	58	59	38	57
Total	100	100	100	100

10. Additional data from physician interviews

10.1 Introduction

This chapter describes some further results of the interview study. The percentage of respondents stating that they have taken a particular decision at some time is first summarised. The distribution according to region (in The Netherlands) and type of institution follows. The position of the nursing staff in MDELs is discussed in Section 10.3. Finally, a possible relation between the interviewers as physicians themselves and the results of the interviews is explored in Section 10.4.

10.2 Various respondents

According to type and specialty

In Chapters 5 to 8 the percentages of physicians practicing particular specialties who had, at some time, taken the MDELs discussed in that particular chapter were presented. This information is summarised in Table 10.1.

There are significant differences between specialties ($P<0.05$, chi-square test)

Table 10.1   Percentages of physicians stating that they have taken some type of MDEL at some time (physician interviews)

	General practitioner n=152 %	Cardio- logist n=34 %	Surgeon n=34 %	Internist n=68 %	Pulmono- logist n=33 %	Neuro- logist n=34 %	Nursing home physician n=50 %	Total n=405 %	p
At some time performed euthanasia or assisted suicide	62	18	35	59	55	32	12	54	< 0.005
At some time performed a life-terminating act without explicit request	30	15	23	26	30	30	10	27	0.07
At some time administered morphine in dosages that almost certainly shortened life	82	68	74	91	94	74	86	82	0.015
At some time withdrawn or withheld treatment upon request (in part) with the purpose of shortening life	45	46	53	41	64	42	53	46	0.28
At some time withdraw or withheld treatment without request	51	75	86	76	90	81	98	62	< 0.005

for three of the five types of MDELs. These differences concern those who have at some time performed euthanasia or assisted suicide, administered morphine at dosages which would possibly shorten life or withdrawn or withheld a treatment without explicit request of the patient.

Table 10.1 allows some conclusions to be drawn. The most important differences are seen in the answers to the first and last questions. More than half of the internists, pulmonologists and general practitioners have, at some time, performed euthanasia or assisted suicide. There is a maximum of 35% for respondents in the other specialties. About half of the general practitioners have at some time withdrawn or withheld treatment without explicit request of the patient. This percentage is much higher for the other groups of physicians. This is obviously a consequence of the different work situations.

There sometimes are considerable differences between clinical specialties. The pulmonologist takes MDELs (considerably) more often than the cardiologist. For the internist and pulmonologist however, there are great similarities between the decision situations.

It is noticeable that only a very small percentage of nursing home physicians state that they have ever performed euthanasia or assisted suicide or have acted without explicit request.

According to region

The provinces of residence are known for all respondents. The provinces were grouped into four regions, as follows:

Groningen, Friesland, Drente: North
Overijssel, Gelderland, Flevoland: East
North- and South-Holland, Utrecht: Randstad
Zeeland, North-Brabant, Limburg: South

Table 10.2 indicates the percentage of physicians stating that they have at some time performed euthanasia or assisted suicide, ranked per region.

The table shows that physicians in the urban agglomeration ("Randstad") performed euthanasia significantly more frequently than those in the other regions. This does not hold for having at some time assisted with suicide. The percentage of physicians in the urban agglomeration that performed euthanasia at some time remains significantly higher than in the other regions of The Netherlands even if the uneven distribution of various types of physicians and specialties in various regions (this analysis is not presented in this book) is taken into account.

Table 10.2   Performed euthanasia or assisted suicide at some time, according to region (physician interviews)

	North n=44 %	East n=80 %	South n=83 %	Randstad n=193 %	Total n=400 %	P
Euthanasia performed at some time	45	41	37	61	50	< 0.005
Assisted suicide performed at some time	9	9	12	12	11	0.84

According to work environment

Specialists and nursing home physicians were asked about the persuasion or policies of the institution of their affilitiation. Comparison of the replies of respondents working in institutions of a particular religious persuasion to replies from those employed in a neutral environment does not indicate a significant difference between the percentages of physicians in the two groups indicating that they have performed euthanasia at some time.

10.3 Nursing staff

Nursing staff were not interviewed in this study, for the reasons discussed in Section 2.2. Much attention was nonetheless given to nursing staff in the course of the physician interviews. Thus the views of physicians about the role of nursing staff in MDELs could be assessed, as well as how these views are reflected in practice.

Several opinions of physicians concerning the tasks of nursing staff were discussed in Section 9.4 and will not be returned to here. There now follows a summary of the information reviewed in Chapters 5 to 7 about consultation with nursing staff about various MDELs.

Table 10.3 presents the percentages of physicians who consulted with nursing staff in connection with a particular decision. In the cases discussed in Chapters 5, 6 and 7 the first question asked was whether nursing staff had been involved with care of the patient. The percentages reported therefore relate to the numbers of cases receiving nursing care.

It is noteworthy that specialists and nursing home physicians almost always had consulted nursing staff in cases of euthanasia, assisted suicide, acting to terminate life without explicit request of the patient and when morphine was administered in high doses so that life would almost certainly be shortened, while

Table 10.3 MDELs taken at some time: consultation with nursing staff by various types of physicians (physician interviews)

	Consultation with nursing staff[1])			
	General practitioner %	Specialist %	Nursing home physician %	Total %
At some time performed euthanasia or assisted suicide (ch.5)	41		96[2])	60
At some time performed a life terminating act without explicit request (ch. 6)	44		98[2])	62
Administered at some time morphine in dosages with almost certain shortening of life (ch.7))	46	98	100	66

1) These percentages refer to cases in which nursing staff was involved with care of the patient.
2) Specialists and nursing home physicians together.

Table 10.4 Role of nursing staff when euthanasia is performed, according to type of physician (physician interviews)

	General practitioner n=152 %	Specialist n=202 %	Nursing home physician n=50 %	Total n=404 %
Euthanasia may only be performed by a physician: % 'in complete agreement' + % 'agree more than disagree'	91	90	88	91
Should nursing staff be permitted to perform the act of euthanasia? − no, never	94	72	92	88

general practitioners consulted nursing staff in fewer than half of cases in which nursing had been involved.

Physicians were also asked if they felt that only a physician may perform euthanasia. Table 10.4 shows that an average of 91% of physicians answered in the affirmative. A discrepancy becomes apparent when the question is asked in a somewhat different manner. In this case 72% of specialists replied in the negative to the question as to whether nursing staff should be permitted to perform the act of euthanasia.

Table 10.5 Differences between replies of respondents interviewed by physicians and interviewed by non-physicians (physician interviews)

	Respondents interviewed			
	by physician n=355 %	by non-physician n=50 %	Total n=405 %	P
Performed euthanasia or assisted suicide at some time	55	45	54	0.35
Never performed euthanasia but considers this conceivable	33	43	34	0.49
Never performed euthanasia and would never do it	13	12	12	0.58
Performed a life-terminating act at some time without explicit request	28	24	27	0.65
Administered morphine or morphine-like drugs in doses that almost certainly shortened life	80	91	82	0.12

10.4 Interviewers

Physicians were mostly used as interviewers in the investigation of Medical Decisions concerning the End of Life. The reasons were given in Section 4.3. Five interviewers who were not physicians were used in addition to 30 physicians.

Table 10.5 compares the results obtained by physician interviewers and non-physician interviewers. The small differences in the table are not statistically significant ($P>0.05$, chi-square test). There also is no relationship between the number of respondents answering the questions of Table 10.5 in the affirmative and the age and sex of the interviewer.

PART III

DEATH CERTIFICATE STUDY

11. Structure of the standard questionnaire

11.1 Introduction

Chapters 11 (Sections 11.1 and 11.2), 12 and 13 were written as the joint responsibility of investigators of the Erasmus University Rotterdam and the Central Bureau of Statistics in The Hague. These chapters describe the development of the standard questionnaire, the design and carrying out of the death certificate study and the results obtained. A detailed description of design, methods and results of this part of the study appeared in the CBS publication "The end of life in medical practice; findings of a survey sampled from deaths occurring July–November 1990" [3].

There were two main directions in the entire investigation (Section 2.3).

The verbal approach to several physicians was the first. The interview questionnaire was used for most of the physicians thus approached (part-study 1), while a more open style of interviewing was used for a small number of experts in a particular area (see Chapter 16).

The second main direction entailed the collection, in writing, of information about deceased individuals. On the one hand, a sample was taken from all deaths known to the CBS for a certain period of time (the death certificate study, part-study 2). On the other hand, physicians who had participated in the interviews were asked to collect, during a period of six months, information in writing on a questionnaire about all deceased patients for whom they had been the treating physician (prospective study, part-study 3). The questionnaire used for part-studies 2 and 3 was identical. The categories established for replies in the interviews (part-study 1) for several important questions were the same that appear in the questionnaire to be completed in writing. This involved questions referring to the classification of decisions as described in Chapter 3 on concepts and definitions. The term 'standard questionnaire' is used for the questionnaire to be completed in writing in view of its central position in the entire investigation.

To be useful for this investigation, the standard questionnaire had to meet several criteria:

1. The treating physician had to be able to fill in this questionnaire independently, without further explanations by an interviewer or others.
2. The questionnaire had to be structured so that all relevant concepts discussed in Chapter 3 would be raised in a way such that in first instance the physician but later a lawyer also could recognise the type of decision.
3. The questionnaire had to be concise because here again a strong appeal was made to the willingness of the physicians to cooperate.

Two other important constraints were also to be considered when both developing and using the questionnaire. First of all, it was not possible to use existing instruments for the development of the questionnaire. As far as we know, no one has previously collected information about the entire spectrum of MDELs by means of written questionnaires. Later in the study the questionnaire developed by Van der Wal et al. [25,26] became available. This questionnaire was used as a basis for several questions in the questionnaire designed for the physician interviews, but not for the standard questionnaire.

A second constraint was the lack of time to carry out a systematic preliminary study. Two approaches were followed to deal with this rather serious limitation. First, the possibility was allowed for that the standard questionnaire would be adjusted, based on the earliest experiences. This indeed turned out to be desirable (see Section 12.4). Moreover, the interview study allowed for the possibility of checking the standard questionnaire by considering what some 370 respondents took to be the meaning of the questions asked. The results of this check are described in Section 11.3.

The standard questionnaire is the product of a very intensive collaboration between researchers of the Erasmus University and the Central Bureau of Statistics.

11.2 Design of the standard questionnaire

The complete text of the standard questionnaire is presented in Appendix A. Only some of the questions are reproduced here which are important for the interpretation of the results. It was mentioned in Section 3.3 that the MDELs are classified basically according to replies to four important questions: what did the physician do; what was the intention of the physician in doing this; had the patient requested this action; was the patient able or unable to express his opinion concerning this action?

The action and the intention of the physician

Questions 4 to 7 of the standard questionnaire concern the action and the intention of the physician (Table 11.1).

In line with the subject matter of Chapter 3 the physician's actions are categorised as withholding treatment, withdrawing treatment and administering drugs. Administering drugs can take the character of either intensification of alleviation of pain and/or symptoms by means of morphine or similar drugs or of explicit and purposeful hastening of the end of life. Morphine is sometimes used in the latter case also. Two intentions can be distinguished for the first two courses of action (withholding or withdrawing treatment), i.e. "taking into account the probability that this action will hasten the end of life of the patient" and "with the explicit purpose of hastening the end of life of the patient".

Regarding intensification of alleviation of pain and/or symptoms there is a third category: "in part with the purpose of hastening the end of life". The background for this third category was discussed in Chapter 3.

It is obvious that question 7 occupies a crucial position. This question does not explicitly use the terms euthanasia, assisted suicide or acting to terminate life without request, but was structured in such a manner that, in combination with other answers from the standard questionnaire, it was possible to define the actions taken by the physician in terms of the three courses of action that were described above.

Definitions can be interpreted in a wide variety of ways. This was the most important consideration for not referring explicitly to the three definitions of actions described above. This was confirmed during the interviews. In several instances a respondent gave an example of euthanasia which, according to the existing definition, should not have been classified as euthanasia. In such situations the interviewer always asked the respondent to give another example.

The choice that was made, not to ask for defined concepts, e.g. euthanasia, but to ask about described actions and intentions has important consequences for the interpretation of the results. This approach may lead, in certain cases, to affirmative answers to question 7 (Table 11.1) by physicians who would not wish to consider this particular way of acting as euthanasia, assisted suicide or terminating life without the patient's request. This indeed occurred, as will be described in Section 11.3.

The sequence of questions 4 to 7 was chosen in such a way that a gradation was achieved, from 'lighter' to 'more severe' actions and intentions. Actions mentioned in question 4 (taking into account the probability that the end of life of the patient will be hastened) can be expected to occur frequently in medical practice. This is in contrast to question 7 regarding the prescribing, supplying or administering of drugs with the explicit purpose of hastening the end of life.

This hierarchy was chosen for two reasons. First, this sequence is helpful for the physician who fills in the questionnaire. Second, it thus becomes possible to assign one particular 'most severe' action and intention to each death case. This is very important for the interpretation of the results.

Question 8 concerns the extent of shortening of life due to the action performed (see Table 11.1). The significance of this question was discussed in Section 3.5. It will become apparent that most of the physicians were prepared to offer an estimate here also.

The role of the patient in decision-making

After the physician had replied to questions 4 to 7 he was asked if a possible hastening of the end of life by the above mentioned actions had been discussed with the patient (see question 9 of Table 11.2).

Table 11.1 Standard questionnaire: questions concerning action and intention of the physician (death certificate study)

---

4. Did you or a colleague take one or more of the following actions, or ensure that one of them was taken, <u>taking into account the probability</u> that this action would hasten the end of the patient's life:

(please reply to all three questions, 4a, 4b and 4c)

4a withholding a treatment*?	0 yes
	0 no
4b withdrawing a treatment *?	0 yes
	0 no
4c intensifying the alleviation of pain and/or symptoms using morphine or a comparable drug?	0 yes-> go to question 5
	0 no-> go to question 6

---

5. Was hastening the end of life <u>partly the purpose</u> of the action indicated in question 4c?

0 yes
0 no

---

6. Was death caused by one or more of the following actions, which you or a colleague decided to take <u>with the explicit purpose</u> of hastening the end of life (answer both 6a and 6b)

6a withholding a treatment*?	0 yes
	0 no
6b withdrawing a treatment*?	0 yes
	0 no

---

7. Was death the caused by the use of a drug** prescribed, supplied, or administered by you or a colleague <u>with the explicit purpose</u> of hastening the end of life (or of enabling the patient to end his own life ?

0 yes
0 no

If yes, who administered this drug** (= introduced it into the body)? (tick one or more answers)

0 the patient himself in tha doctor's presence
0 the patient himself without the doctor being present
0 you or a colleague
0 a nurse
0 another person in the doctor's presence
0 another person without the doctor being present

---

8. A question about that (last mentioned) action:
In your estimation, by how much was the life of the patient in fact shortened by this action?

0 more than six months
0 one to six months
0 one to four weeks
0 up to one week
0 less than 24 hours
0 life probably was not shortened at all

---

*   In this study, 'treatment' is taken to include 'tube feeding'

**   This may mean one or more drugs; morphine is also sometimes used for this purpose.

Table 11.2   **The most important questions about the role of the patient in decision-taking (death certificate study)**

9. Did you or a colleague discuss with the patient the (possible) hastening of the end of life as a result of the last-mentioned action?	0 yes, at the time of performing the action or shortly before –> go to question 10 0 yes, some time beforehand (and not at the time of, or shortly before) –> go to question 10 0 yes, I do not know when – > go to question 10 0 no, no discussion -> go to question 16
12. Was the decision concerning the (last-mentioned) action taken upon an explicit request of the patient?	0 yes -> go to question 13 0 no -> go to question 15
13. At the time of this request, did you consider the patient able to assess his/her situation and take a decision about it adequately?	0 yes 0 no, not or not totally able
16. Was it possible to discuss the situation with the patient at the time when the (last-mentioned) action was decided upon?	0 yes 0 no
17. Why was this decision not discussed with the patient? (tick one or more answers)	0 patient was too young 0 patient was too emotionally unstable 0 this (last-mentioned) action was clearly the best one for the patient 0 discussion would have done more harm than good 0 patient was temporarily unconscious 0 patient was permanently unconscious 0 patient was in a state of diminished consciousness 0 patient was demented 0 patient was mentally handicapped 0 patient was suffering from a psychiatric disorder 0 others, if you wish you may expand on this at question 24
19. As far as you know, had the patient ever express a wish for the end of life to be hastened?	0 yes -> go to question 20 0 no – > go to question 21

If there had been a discussion with the patient, the next question was whether there had been an explicit request of the patient and if the patient, in the opinion of the physician, had been able to assess the situation and take a decision adequately.

If the physician replied that there had not been any discussion, he was asked if it would have been possible to discuss this matter with the patient (question 16) and why there had not been any discussion (question 17). It was also asked (question 19) if the patient had ever indicated his wishes as to hastening the end of life.

The standard questionnaire contained a total of 24 questions which, together with other available background information, permitted a large number of detailed analyses. In order that the main argument of this book be followed it was necessary to introduce several reductions from the very beginning. The most important reduction concerned questions 4 to 7. It was possible to reply affirmatively to several of these questions for one particular death case. If a physician indicated to have withheld a treatment with the explicit purpose of shortening life (yes to question 6a) it is logical that the physician also considered the probability that life would be shortened by this action (yes to question 4a). In most cases in which questions 6a or 6b were answered affirmatively this indeed was also the case for questions 4a and 4b. The end of life could also have been hastened by a combination of actions such as withholding a treatment, withdrawing treatment and intensifying alleviation of pain and/or symptoms using morphine.

The incidence of the above mentioned combinations will be reported upon in the discussion of the results of the death certificate study and the prospective study. Strong simplification will be applied in the discussion of patient characteristics, decision procedures etc. All deaths will be classified according to the 'last mentioned action' from questions 4 to 7 to which therespondent replied in the affirmative. When, for instance, question 7 was answered by 'yes', the case was classified as belonging to the category 'question 7', regardless of which previous questions might also have been answered in the affirmative.

This is reasonable because the sequence of questions 4 to 7 was chosen so as to build a hierarchy into the possible actions and intentions of the physician.

11.3 Interpretation of questions 4 to 7

It is obviously important to know how respondents have interpreted the questions of the standard questionnaire, particularly questions 4 to 7.

The physician interview study was used to get an impression of their interpretation. All respondents in that study had received a copy of the standard questionnaire prior to the interview. They were asked to fill in the questionnaire for the most recent death they had experienced as treating physician, unless this death had been completely unexpected and sudden. The completed questionnaire was then discussed by interviewer and respondent at the beginning of the interview. This procedure permitted checking of the kind of death concerned and the specific actions taken.

In most instances the respondent had filled in the standard questionnaire prior to the visit of the interviewer. There were cases, when the questionnaire had not been filled in and in situations when only a very limited amount of time was available, in which this questionnaire was not discussed. A total of 370 questionnaires were discussed between interviewer and respondent, with particular emphasis on questions 4 to 7. The results are presented in Appendix D and are reviewed briefly below.

The respondents supplied important new information about the interpretation of the questions of the standard questionnaire in 29 of 370 cases. In all other cases, the relation between the case described by the respondent and the information filled in on the standard questionnaire was clear. The 29 cases mostly involved a shift towards a less 'serious' intention with respect to the category of action indicated.

It is of particular importance that 9 out of 34 respondents who answered question 7 affirmatively subsequently commented on this confirming answer. Intensification of alleviation of pain and/or symptoms with morphine was involved in several cases and the respondent felt that "in part with the purpose to accelerate the end of life" was a better description of his intention than "with the explicit purpose". In some other cases the respondent indicated that neither euthanasia, assisted suicide nor terminating life were at issue, in spite of an affirmative answer to question 7. The following case description is a good example:

A patient in the last phase of cancer develops pneumonia. After discussion with the patient therapy of the pneumonia is not initiated. The patient continues to receive morphine against pain. The patient dies 30 hours later. The respondent estimates that the life of the patient was shortened by two weeks because of not administering antibiotics and by 24 hours due to morphine.

Patient and physician had discussed euthanasia earlier and had decided against it.

This case is an example of several case descriptions in which, in the opinion of the respondents, it would have been more correct to record question 6 rather than question 7 as the last-mentioned MDEL-action. Other cases involved the administration of exclusively morphine in a terminal stage of the disease. These respondents felt that their cases definitely did not belong to the category of euthanasia and therefore were not suitable for further questioning in that part of the interview that dealt with euthanasia.

This situation was also encountered in the death certificate study. In a small number of cases the comment that had been written on the questionnaire was reason to change the reply to question 7 into 'no'. Moreover, several respondents felt that the distinction between questions 5 and 7 was very difficult.

Two important factors played a role in the interpretation of question 6.

The first was that in several cases the patient explicitly refused therapy or wished to have therapy stopped, against the advice of the physician. In such cases it is not possible to consider this as an action the physician decided upon to hasten the end of life.

A second important point is that, in several cases, the respondent reported that he had decided not to prolong the patient's life. This important matter was discussed in Section 3.5. This distinction did not play an important role in either the death certificate study or the prospective study. Only in a small number of cases did the respondent indicate on the questionnaire that he wished to make a distinction between "forego prolongation of life" and "hasten the end of life".

These findings have two important consequences for the interpretation of the results of the death certificate study and the prospective study. The first consequence is that, in the opinion of the respondent, affirmative replies to question 7 must not merely be interpreted as euthanasia, assisted suicide or performing a life-terminating act without explicit request, but must receive further consideration. In several cases the situation is that only morphine was administered and the life of the dying patient was shortened by only a brief period. Considering the affirmative replies to question 7, such actions are considered as very "serious" by respondents, but not as euthanasia, assisted suicide or performing a life-terminating act without explicit request.

A second conclusion is that several affirmative replies to questions 6a and 6b refer to situations in which the patient refused further therapy without the physician's participation in this decision and to several situations in which the physician foregoes the possibility of a limited prolongation of life.

12. Design and carrying out of the death certificate study

12.1 Introduction

When working on the design of this study it was clear from the beginning that drawing a sample of physicians would not be sufficient for arriving at good quantitative estimates. A large sample drawn from a great number of deaths would also be necessary for a solidly based estimate. There are two places where data concerning deaths are assembled; the population registers of the municipalities and the Central Bureau of Statistics (CBS) where data for deaths of all Dutch residents are collected. The CBS receives on the one hand personal data regarding the deceased and on the other hand the death certificate completed by the physician (the ''B'' form). Thus the CBS is the ideal basis for drawing a sample of deaths. The CBS was therefore invited in the beginning of 1990 to participate in study 2, the death certificate study, to be performed in close collaboration with the investigators of the Erasmus University.

The investigators of the CBS developed within a short period of time a design in which sample taking, procedures to ensure anonymity etc. were detailed. Investigators from the two institutions together developed the standard questionnaire (see Chapter 11).

The design of the death certificate study will be discussed in the remainder of this chapter.

12.2 Drawing a sample

The CBS department for cause-of-death statistics receives a medical death certificate, the B form. This certificate is anonymous with respect to the person deceased. It contains some concise personal data as well as the cause of death. The certificate is filled in by the treating physician, the physician on call or locum or the coroner. The certificates, the contents of which are kept secret, are processed by the municipal administration and mailed monthly to the CBS. These declarations are the material from which the samples were drawn.

The size of the sample was 8500 deaths. The procedure of drawing samples was stratified, which made it possible to obtain more reliable information with the same size of the sample.

Each B form arriving at the CBS was looked at by a physician and assigned to one of five previously defined groups, the strata. A higher stratum number suggests a greater chance of an MDEL relevant for the study. For stratum 0 this chance is almost nil because the death certificate shows that no medical acts were involved and certainly no acts that would shorten life. In stratum 1 the chance is small but not nil, in stratum 2 there is a possibility, in stratum 3 a serious chance and in stratum 4 the chance is great, all of this based on information recorded by the treating physician on the B form. The required elements for the sample were drawn from each stratum. Death assigned to a stratum with a higher number had a greater chance of being drawn.

The treating physician was contacted (as far as possible) for each of the elements drawn in groups 1 to 4. In most cases this was the person signing the B form or the treating physician who could be found with the cooperation of the signing physician. The treating physician received the standard questionnaire together with an accompanying letter from the physician charged with causes-of-death statistics and a supporting letter from the Chief Inspector of the Health Supervisory Service and the Chairman of the KNMG. No standard questionnaire needed to be mailed for cases of stratum 0 because it was clear that in such cases no MDEL was taken.

12.3 Anonymity guarantee

Considering the sensitivity of the topic it was of utmost importance to develop a procedure that would guarantee absolute anonymity of both physician and deceased. It had to be possible to guarantee that nobody would be able to trace either the respondent who had filled in the questionnaire or the deceased who was the subject of the questionnaire, from the moment the filled-in questionnaire was returned to the time of its processing by the CBS.

Therefore a unique procedure was developed for the CBS to achieve this anonymity.

Participating physicians returned the filled-in questionnaires to a notary instead of directly to the CBS. The questionnaires were in a closed envelope under a number that was meaningless for the notary. Based on this number the notary added some details taken from the information on the B form that could not serve to identify anyone: background data and stratum number. Thereafter the notary removed the above mentioned number from the envelope and forwarded the number to the CBS. CBS staff removed all data recorded under the particular number from all files in such a manner that no reconstruction was possible. Only after the protocol for this removal of data had been presented to the notary did the latter hand over the now totally anonymous envelopes to the CBS. This procedure guaranteed complete anonymity: neither notary nor CBS had information that would allow the completed questionnaires to be traced to specific death cases or physicians.

The background data mentioned above concerned sex, age (in 7 categories), cause of death (12 categories) and the place of death (hospital/elsewhere). The possible number of combinations of age and cause of death was reduced to 55, which excluded the possibility of tracing the individual based on the combination of age and cause of death.

The information available for each deceased in the death certificate study thus consisted of background data, stratum number and filled-in standard questionnaire.

12.4 Carrying out the study

The population studied consisted of all deaths for the months of July up to (and including) November 1990. The death certificates for these cases reached the CBS in the period from August 1990 up to (and including) February 1991. Two physicians and two temporary administrators were employed to inspect and process 50 000 B forms, under the close guidance of the staff of the CBS Departments of Health Statistics and of Statistical Methods. A number of elements (8500 or 17%) drawn from these forms represented the sample. A standard questionnaire was mailed to respondents in more than 8000 cases; in some 350 cases the deceased was classified as stratum 0 and no questionnaire needed to be dispatched. Some 100 elements were not sent out, mainly because the physician concerned could not be traced.

The results obtained from several test interviews and from the first filled-in standard questionnaires made it necessary to introduce some modifications in the standard questionnaire. This meant that the standard questionnaire used for the July deaths was slightly different from the questionnaire used for subsequent months. To ensure consistency only results for the months August to November 1990 will be presented, representing a total of 41 587 deaths. However, no major differences were found when comparisons could be made between July and the remaining months. The CBS report discusses this "July response" in more detail [3].

12.5 Response and representativeness

Response

Of the standard questionnaires mailed to respondents, 76% were returned. The reasons for non-return of the remaining 24% could not be elucidated in view of the absolute anonymity enforced. It is almost certain that there were involved not only refusal to participate but various technical causes for non-return such as questionnaires not reaching their destination, treating physician no longer to be found, etc. The response in the death certificate study was 73% after removal of questionnaires that could not be processed and application of several other corrections. This percentage (73%) takes into account the differences in sample fraction per stratum mentioned earlier. This response percentage can be considered as relatively high considering the fact that physicians had been asked to provide confidential information voluntarily some time after the patient had died and had to make a considerable amount of time available. We assume that the careful presentation to the medical profession, the recommendation by the Chief Inspector of the Health Supervisory Service and the Chairman of the Royal Dutch Medical Association played an important role in this willingness to respond.

It is noteworthy that the percentage of responses hardly differed whether the filled-in questionnaires were subdivided according to stratum, sex, age or group of diagnosis. Only in a few small groups of patients (lower age, rare cause of death) were the deviations from the average sometimes slightly larger. However, this also could have been a matter of chance and need not be taken as pointing to a systematic difference in response behaviour. There is an important difference only when a distinction is made according to the place of death. The response rate was 64% for deaths that occurred in hospital while this percentage for other places was 81%. There are, however, no differences between age, sex and cause of death within each of these two groups. There also were no differences according to stratum. This means that bias of the results due to selectivity among the non-responses, although it can never be totally excluded, is not likely. The distribution of the responses according to sex, age, group of diagnosis, place of death and number of stratum is presented in Appendix C.

Weighting procedure

A weighting procedure was applied for the derivation of estimates valid for the whole population of deceased persons that takes into account differences between sampling fraction and response percentages. The weights were derived after subdivision of the sample according to place of death, cause of death, age and sex. A further adjustment was made to bring the distribution of the weighted estimates according to age and sex in line with the age and sex distribution of the whole population of The Netherlands. A small error may remain because the distribution according to place and cause of death depended on the chance result of sampling. The weighting procedure is discussed in more detail in Appendix E.

The quality of the data

The quality of the data obtained is determined by a great many factors, such as:

- clarity of the standard questionnaire;
- the ability of the respondent to recall the death case or trace the information required;
- the meticulousness of the physician in filling in the questionnaire.

In spite of the difficulty of the topic and the demands made on the respondent the quality of the filled-in questionnaires was, on the whole, very good. The care the physicians devoted to filling in the questionnaires was evidenced in many ways. On a large number of questionnaires additional information was presented to clarify the choice of answers made. In some instances this information made it possible to correct the distribution of the replies to the questions in the questionnaire. In the great majority of cases, however, the additional information confirmed the replies given in the questionnaire.

Moreover, the quality of the replies became apparent from the internal consistency of the replies. The researchers of the CBS and the Erasmus University jointly produced rules regarding decisions that permitted consistency to be ascertained and inconsistencies to be resolved. The solutions were almost always obvious and in the majority of cases the replies were entirely consistent. It was eventually concluded that some 2% of the replies contained information that could not be used. This often concerned situations in which the respondent did not know whether important decisions concerning the particular end of life had been taken (e.g. locum during evening hours). There also were questionnaires that had been returned directly to the CBS. These directly returned questionnaires did not have an element number so that stratum number and background data could not be added (see Section 12.3).

The accuracy of the results of the different component studies is discussed in Chapter 17 and Appendix E.

13. Results of the death certificate study

13.1 Introduction

The results of the death certificate study are presented in this chapter. Similarly to the physician interview study, the decision was made not to present too many details in this case also. This was necessary in order to allow the reader to keep a grasp on the entire project and to follow the main argument from definition of the problem to discussion of the results. This decision implies that several interesting details are not covered in this book. The reader is again referred to the separate report of the Central Bureau of Statistics [3] for further details. The results presented in this chapter are based on the deaths during the period from August to November 1990 and thus are, strictly speaking, valid only for that period.

13.2 Occurrence of MDELs

The structure of the standard questionnaire was discussed in Chapter 11. Questions 4 to 7 of the standard questionnaire concern the act and the intention of the physician. The formulation of these questions can be found in Table 11.1 and in the standard questionnaire presented in Appendix A. The actions and intentions described in these questions are summarised in the present chapter as the 'MDEL-action' concept. MDEL-actions are, therefore, defined as combinations of an action and an intention:

- withholding or withdrawing treatment, taking into account the probability that this action will hasten the end of life of the patient or with the explicit purpose of hastening the end of life;
- intensifying of alleviation of pain and/or symptoms taking into account the probability that this action will hasten the end of life or in part with the purpose of hastening the end of life of the patient;
- prescribing, supplying or administering drugs with the explicit purpose of hastening the end of life.

An MDEL-action is taken to have been performed if one or more of questions 4 to 7 was answered in the affirmative.

Table 13.1 shows the distribution of the various MDEL-actions over the death cases. The first column shows the percentage of affirmative answers to the particular question. This information cannot be interpreted in isolation, without further details because in several cases more than one MDEL-action was performed in a patient.

Table 13.1   MDEL-actions performed by the physician (death certificate study)

	Replies given total n')= 5197 %³)	of which as last mentioned MDEL-action n')= 5197 %
No MDEL-action performed	**60,6**	**60,6**
stratum 0²)	9.0	9.0
First contact after the death (excluding stratum 0)	2.8	2.8
Sudden and totally unexpected death (excluding stratum 0)	18.1	18.1
Other cases where no MDEL-action was performed (no 'yes' to questions 4 to 7) (excluding stratum 0)	30.6	30.6
MDEL-action performed	**39.4**	**39.4**
Taking into account the probability that the end of life was hastened by		
4a withholding a treatment	21.6	5.6
4b withdrawing a treatment	13.9	3.6
4c intensifying alleviation of pain and/or symptoms	25.0	15.0
In part with the purpose of hastening the end of life by		
5 intensifying alleviation of pain and/or symptoms	7.6	3.8
With the explicit purpose of hastening the end of life by:		
6a withholding a treatment	7.1	4.3
6b withdrawing a treatment	5.1	4.3
7 prescribing, supplying or administering a drug	2.7	2.7
Total	**100.0**	**100.0**

1)   Total number of standard questionnaires with a usable response on which this column is based, plus stratum 0.

2)   Because no standard questionnaires had been sent of stratum 0, the distribution over the next three categories is not known. It is known, however, that no MDEL-action was performed in these cases (see section 12.2 and the text of the standard questionnaire).

3)   The percentages in this column add up to more than 100%, because more than one of questions 4 to 7 could be answered with "yes".

It is particularly important for this study to decide which was the most serious MDEL-action. The structure of the standard questionnaire was such that the last affirmative reply (yes) to questions 4 to 7 could generally be considered as the most serious MDEL-action (see Section 11.2). The last affirmative answer was determined for each death for which at least one of questions 4 to 7 was answered affirmatively. The distribution of these 'last-mentioned MDEL-actions' is presented in the second column of Table 13.1.

The data presented here show that no MDEL-action was performed for 60.6% of the deceased. Sudden and totally unexpected death occurred in 18% of cases and death was not sudden but no MDEL-action was performed in 31%. In 12% of the cases (stratum 0 or first contact after death had occurred) it was unknown whether death had occurred suddenly. An MDEL-action was performed in 39.4% of deceased patients.

The largest single category of MDEL-actions is that of intensifying alleviation of pain and/or symptoms, taking into account the probability that this will hasten the end of life (15.0% ''yes'' to question 4c). Intensification of alleviation of pain and/or symptoms with in part the purpose of hastening the end of life (last ''yes'' to question 5) occurred in 3.8% of cases. When withholding or withdrawing treatment are combined, this occurred in 17.9% of all cases as the last-mentioned MDEL-action (last ''yes'' to questions 4a, 4b, 6a or 6b).

In half of these cases the explicit purpose was to hasten the end of life (last ''yes'' to questions 6a or 6b).

It should be emphasised once more that that the explicit purpose of hastening the end of life was derived from the explicit purpose of reducing or ending suffering.

The physician indicated in 2.7% of cases that death was the consequence of the use of a drug prescribed, supplied or administered by himself or a colleague with the explicit purpose of hastening the end of life or enabling the patient himself to end his life (''yes'' in question 7).

13.3 Extent of shortening of life

The standard questionnaire contains a question as to the respondent's estimate of the amount of time by which the life of the patient was shortened by the action mentioned last in the questionnaire. Table 13.2 presents a summary of the extents to which the patient's life was shortened in the opinion of the respondent. The table provides an impression of the relative weight of the various last-mentioned actions. However, it should be mentioned that 11% of respondents did not supply information about the extent of shortening of life. This lack of information is particularly clustered around cases in which the last-mentioned MDEL-action was that indicated by the response to question 4.

It is obvious that in most instances there was no shortening of life when the answer to one of questions 4a, 4b or 4c indicated the last-mentioned MDEL-action. It seems that an actual effect was not considered present although there was the probability that the life of the patient would be shortened by this action. A shortening of life did occur, in the opinion of the physician, in most of the cases for which questions 5 to 7 were answered affirmatively. At the other end of the spectrum are situations in which there was shortening of life by more than half a year. The table shows that this concerns about 1% of cases. In general, life was shortened by a maximum of one week in 75% of the cases. Life shortening was more than one week in about 15% of cases. This more serious

Table 13.2   Extent of shortening of life, based on last mentioned MDEL-action (death certificate study)

	Last-mentioned MDEL-action[1])							
	4a n= 309 %	4b n= 204 %	4c n= 922 %	5 n= 244 %	6a n= 244 %	6b n= 234 %	7 n= 204 %	Total n= 2361 %
Unknown	13	17	17	2	5	3	1	11
no shortening	46	48	48	12	16	12	1	34
<24 hours	5	11	16	35	7	20	24	16
1 day to 1 week	17	13	14	41	35	46	41	25
1 to 4 weeks	11	8	4	9	24	14	19	10
1 to 6 months	7	2	2	1	10	3	11	4
>1/2 year	1	0	0	–	3	1	3	1
Total	100	100	100	100	100	100	100	100

1)   Taking into account the probability that the end of life was hastened by:
 4a withholding a treatment
 4b withdrawing a treatment
 4c intensifying alleviation of pain and/or symptoms
In part with the purpose of hastening the end of life by:
 5 intensifying alleviation of pain and/or symptoms
With the explicit purpose of hastening the end of life by:
 6a withholding a treatment
 6b withdrawing a treatment
 7 prescribing, supplying or administering a drug

shortening of life is unevenly distributed over various types of MDEL-actions. In cases where question 7 was answered in the affirmative, life was shortened by more than one week in one third of the cases. This is also true for the cases for which it was decided to withhold a treatment with the explicit purpose of hastening the end of life (question 6a).

Two important conclusions can be drawn from the table. First, there is an important difference between the extent of shortening of life due to actions implied in question 4 and those implied in questions 5 to 7. Second, withholding a treatment can be a weighty medical decision that can have the same effect as administering, prescribing or supplying of drugs with the explicit purpose of hastening the end of life.

13.4 Role of the patient in 'decision-taking'

The standard questionnaire contains several questions about the role of the patient when a decision was taken (see Section 11.2). The key question here is question 9: ''Was the last-mentioned MDEL-action discussed with the patient?''.

The answers to question 9 are summarised in Table 13.3, subdivided according to various last-mentioned MDEL-actions.

The most important finding was that when question 7 was answered affirmatively, this had been discussed with the patient in 83% of cases. In the other MDEL-actions there was no discussion with the patient in 60% of cases. There are, however, differences. When question 5 was answered affirmatively discussion had taken place in more than half the cases.

Withholding or withdrawing treatment treatment was not discussed with the patient in two thirds of the cases.

13.5 Decision-taking in discussion with the patient

Table 13.4 provides further information about the taking of a decision when the action concerned was discussed with the patient. For the sake of clarity the MDEL-actions referred to in questions 4a and 4b were combined in table 13.4 and following tables. This was also done with questions 6a and 6b. This was justified because most of the aspects to be discussed regarding withdrawing treatment or withholding treatment with the same intention show important similarities.

Table 13.3 Discussion with the patient about the decision to be taken, according to "last-mentioned" MDEL-action (death certificate study)

	Last-mentioned MDEL-action[1]							Total with MDEL-action
	4a n= 309 %	4b n= 204 %	4c n= 922 %	5 n= 244 %	6a n= 244 %	6b n= 234 %	7 n= 204 %	n= 2361 %
Discussed	27	19	30	53	33	39	83	36
Not discussed	63	67	52	45	64	59	17	54
Unknown	9	14	18	2	3	2	–	10
Total	100	100	100	100	100	100	100	100

1) Taking into account the probability that the end of life was hastened by:
    4a withholding a treatment
    4b withdrawing a treatment
    4c intensifying alleviation of pain and/or symptoms
    In part with the purpose of hastening the end of life by:
    5   intensifying alleviation of pain and/or symptoms
    With the explicit purpose of hastening the end of life by:
    6a withholding a treatment
    6b withdrawing a treatment
    7   prescribing, supplying or administering a drug

Table 13.4 Decision-taking after discussion with the patient, according to last-mentioned MDEL-action (death certificate study)

	4a/b n=136 %	4c n= 291 %	5 n=134 %	6a/6b n= 185 %	7 n=179 %	Total n= 925 %
Last-mentioned MDEL-action [1] [2]						
Decision taken upon explicit request						
by patient	52	48	53	63	84	59
Explicit and repeated request	47	38	49	55	79	51
Written advance directive	3	3	10	6	42	11
Patient totally able to take a decision	83	84	84	75	96	84
Initiative for discussion came from [3]:						
− patient	41	39	58	46	74	49
− physician (and not from patient)	54	56	32	49	21	54
In addition to discussion with patient there was discussion with [3]:						
− colleagues	57	58	60	62	81	63
− nursing staff	47	49	59	64	40	52
− relatives	65	70	77	82	87	76
− no one	9	8	5	2	2	6

1) Percentages in this table always refer to the total number of patients per last-mentioned action with whom this action had been discussed
2) Taking into account the probability that the end of life was hastened by:
    4a/b withholding or withdrawing a treatment
    4c intensifying alleviation of pain and/or symptoms
  In part with the purpose to hasten the end of life by:
    5 intensifying alleviation of pain and/or symptoms.
  With the explicit purpose of hastening the end of life by:
    6a/b withholding and/or withdrawing a treatment ;
    7 prescribing, supplying or administering a drug
3) More than one answer could be given to this question.

The first line of Table 13.4 shows that the action was performed upon explicit request of the patient in more than half of the cases if a consultation with the patient had taken place about a last-mentioned MDEL-action. This holds in particular for the actions referred to in questions 6 and 7. In approximately half the cases the initiative for a consultation came from the patient. When question 7 was answered affirmatively, this percentage was 74%. The physician took the initiative for a consultation about an action as referred to in question 7 in 21% of cases.

When a consultation between physician and patient had taken place we know whether at the time of the consultation, the patient was capable to assess his situation and take a decision adequately. In addition, an assessment of the particular patient was available in the case that an explicit request had been made. We gave this last assessment particular weight when the question as to the patient's capability to assess the situation had to be decided. However, it hardly ever happened that the physician considered the patient capable to assess his situation during the consultation and no longer capable when making the explicit request. Of the patients with whom a consultation took place 84% were completely capable of assessing their situation. This holds for almost all cases with an affirmatively reply to question 7.

A written advance declaration was available in 42% of the cases for whom question 7 was replied to affirmatively and a consultation had taken place. This was only exceptionally the case for all other MDEL-actions.

A colleague was consulted about the last-mentioned MDEL-action in more than half the cases in which a consultation with the patient had taken place. When a MDEL-action as referred to in question 7 was concerned, a colleague was consulted in 81% of cases.

13.6 Decision-taking without discussion with the patient

It was not discussed with the patient in 54% of cases (Table 13.3). The MDEL-action of question 7 was not discussed with the patient in 17% of cases. Some characteristics of decision-taking without discussion with the patient are presented in Table 13.5.

The first row of table 13.5 shows that in 86% of the cases in which no discussion with the patient had taken place the opinion of the physician was that this had not been possible. In all affirmative replies to question 7 which state that no discussion with the patient had taken place it is also mentioned that, in the opinion of the physician, this had not been possible.

Two questions were available to classify the cases in which there was no discussion between physician and patient according to the patient's ability to take a decision: the question as to the reason(s) why there had not been any discussion with the patient (question 17) and the question as to whether discussion would have been possible (question 16). A division was made according to whether the patients were "able" and "not able" to take a decision.

All patients with whom had not been discussed for one or more of the following reasons: permanently unconscious, temporarily unconscious, mentally handicapped and too young were classified as 'not able to take a decision'. These reasons made discussion impossible, with the exception of very few cases. Moreover, if no discussion had been possible patients with reduced consciousness or dementia were classified as unable to take a decision. All other combinations

134

of answers to questions 16 and 17 were classified as 'ability to take decisions unknown'. This included among others answers such as "patient emotionally too labile", "clearly the best for the patient" and "discussion would have done more harm than good", not combined with other categories of answers. Intensifying alleviation of pain and/or symptoms was often involved in these cases. The reasons for not discussing with the patient are presented in Table 13.6.

Returning to Table 13.5 after this discussion about the ability of patients to take a decision it appears that 81% of patients with whom had not been discussed could not have been discused with because of their inability to take a decision.

Table 13.5 **Decision-taking without discussing with the patient, according to last-mentioned MDEL-action[1]) (death certificate study)**

	Last-mentioned MDEL-action[2])					
	4a/b n= 321 %	4c n= 468 %	5 n=105 %	6a/b n= 282 %	7 n= 25 %	Total n=1201 %
No discussion possible	91	77	88	94	100	86
Patient unable to take a decision	87	72	77	88	85	81
Patient had at some time indicated a wish to hasten the end of life	11	9	22	16	25	13
An explicit request to hasten the end of life of patient by:						
− relatives	7	8	25	26	49	14
− physician/nurse/others (but not relatives)	0	1	1	2	3	1
− no one	84	84	70	67	49	78
Decision discussed with [3]):						
− colleagues	42	31	43	53	70	42
− nursing staff	55	36	58	66	79	51
− relatives	68	52	70	81	87	66
− no one	16	29	15	5	3	18

1) The percentages in this table always refer to the total number of patients per last-mentioned action with whom the action had not been discussed.
2) Taking into account the probability that the end of life was hastened by:
    4a/b withholding and/or withdrawing a treatment
    4c intensifying alleviation of pain and/or symptoms
  In part with the purpose of hastening the end of life by:
    5 intensifying alleviation of pain and/or symptoms
  With the explicit purpose of hastening the end of life by:
    6a/b withholding and/or withdrawing a treatment
    7 prescribing, supplying or administering a drug.
3) More than one answer coud be given to this question.

Table 13.6 Reasons for not discussing with the patient, according to last-mentioned MDEL-action[1]) (death certificate study)

	Last-mentioned MDEL-action[2])					
	4a/b n= 321 %	4c n= 468 %	5 n=105 %	6a/b n= 282 %	7 n= 25 %	Total n=1201 %
Too young	2	1	1	4	9	2
Emotionally too labile (b)	1	2	5	1	3	2
Clearly the best for the patient (c)	11	28	27	14	26	20
Would have done more harm than good (d)	6	6	11	6	0	6
Only b and/or c and/or d and no other answering category (ability to take a decision not known)	7	17	18	6	8	11
Temporarily unconscious	4	3	1	5	–	4
Permanently unconscious	27	12	11	24	23	19
Reduced consciousness	39	46	57	42	57	44
Demented	32	22	23	32	11	27
Mentally handicapped	1	2	1	1	–	1
Mental disorder	5	2	–	2	3	2
Other reason	2	3	2	3	5	3
Unknown	4	6	4	2	8	4

1) More than one answer could be given to this question

2) Taking into account the probability that the end of life was hastened by:
  4a/b withholding and/or withdrawing a treatment
  4c intensifying alleviation of pain and/or symptoms
  In part with the purpose of hastening the end of life by
  5 intensifying alleviation of pain and/or symptoms
  With the explicit purpose of hastening the end of life by:
  6a/b withholding and/or withdrawing a treatment
  7 prescribing, supplying or administering a drug.

Some of the patients with whom had not been discussed had previously expressed a desire to have their life shortened. This occurs more frequently with respect to the more weighty actions (questions 5 to 7).

Table 13.5 also shows the fraction of cases in which others than the patient had made an explicit request to hasten the end of life of the patient. In total, relatives had made such an explicit request in 14% of cases and others had made the request in 1%. An explicit request by relatives occurs most often when more weighty MDEL-actions are involved. This occurs in about one quarter of cases with respect to MDEL-actions associated with questions 5 and 6 , and in almost half the number of cases for question 7.

Consultation with colleagues occurred less often when it had not been discussed with the patient than when there had been discussion (Tables 13.4 and 13.5). Nursing staff was consulted in about half the cases, regardless of whether there had or had not been a discussion with the patient. There is a difference, however, if question 7 was answered in the affirmative. If there was no discussion with the patient, there was in most cases consultation with the nursing staff.

13.7 Distribution according to age, sex, cause of death and type of physician

The 'last-mentioned' MDEL-actions associated with questions 4 to 7 are subdivided according to age, sex, several causes of death and specialty in Tables 13.7 to 13.9. In Tables 13.7 and 13.8 the percentages are presented in two ways. The first two columns of the table show the percentage of cases for which at least one of questions 4 to 7 was answered affirmatively, for each separate class of the particular category (e.g. a particular age group). The next five columns show the distribution of the particular characteristic over the various classes for each separate last-mentioned MDEL-action. The last column gives the distribution of the total number of deaths in The Netherlands in the same form.

Age

In Table 13.7 it is noteworthy that the percentage of death cases for which at least one of questions 4 to 7 was answered affirmatively differs only slightly between the four age groups. Only in the youngest age group is the percentage of death cases with an MDEL-action a little lower, 32%, than the average, 39%. This value for the highest age group is 42%.

There are, however, important differences between the distribution of 'last-mentioned' MDEL-actions between the age groups. Decisions to withhold or withdraw a treatment occur relatively more often in the highest age group. The decision to intensify alleviation of pain and/or symptoms occurs more often in the group 65 to 79 years of age. The actions implied in question 7 occur relatively often in age groups up to 64 years.

Sex

The distribution beween sexes also shows several differences (Table 13.7). There was no MDEL-action for 57% of women who died, while this percentage was 64% for men. The most noticeable finding was that the MDEL-action referred to by question 7 occurs more often with men than women. All other MDEL-actions occur more often with women. There is, however, a relationship between sex and average age at death, this age being considerably higher for

Table 13.7 Age and sex, according to last-mentioned MDEL-action (death certificate study)

	MDEL-action	No MDEL-action	Last-mentioned MDEL-action[1]					together	All actions 1990[2]	Mortality in The Netherl.
			4a/b n=513	4c n=922	5 n=244	6a/b n=478	7 n=204	n=2361	n=128786
	%[3]	%[3]	%	%	%	%	%	%	%
% last-mentioned action	39	61	9	15	4	9	3	39	
Age									
0-49	32	68	5	6	6	9	14	7	8
50-64	40	60	9	16	21	9	24	14	13
65-79	38	62	31	40	41	32	38	36	37
80+	42	58	56	38	32	50	25	43	42
Total	39	61	100	100	100	100	100	100	100
Sex									
Male	36	64	46	48	48	45	61	48	52
Female	43	57	54	52	52	55	39	52	48
Total	39	61	100	100	100	100	100	100	100

1) Taking into account the probability that the end of life was hastened by:
    4a/b withholding and/or withdrawing a treatment
    4c intensifying alleviation of pain and/or symptoms
In part with the purpose of hastening the end of life by:
    5 intensifying alleviation of pain and/or symptoms
With the explicit purpose of hastening the end of life by:
    6a/b withholding and/or withdrawing a treatment
    7 prescribing, supplying or administering a drug.
2) Source: CBS causes-of-death statistics
3) Row percentages

women than for men. To discuss this in more detail would go beyond the scope of this book.

Cause of death

The distribution of causes of death, shown in Table 13.8, also shows marked differences. In deaths due to cancer, an MDEL-action was performed in 60% of cases. At the other extreme are the external causes (accidents, poisonings, violence), in which an MDEL-action was performed in 12% of cases. The incidence of MDEL-actions was also limited, 21% of cases, in cardiovascular illnesses.

If the distribution of MDEL-actions over the groups for causes of death is considered, it becomes clear that in more than half the cases intensifying of alleviation of pain and/or symptoms and administering, supplying or prescribing of drugs with the explicit purpose of hastening the end of life concerns patients suffering from cancer. In this respect it should be kept in mind that cancer is the most important cause of death (27% of all deaths) in The Netherlands.

Decisions related to withdrawing or withholding treatment (questions 4a and 4b and 6a and 6b) are much more widely spread over several cause-of-death groups; diseases of the nervous system are relatively strongly represented.

Type of physician

Table 13.9 presents the distribution over the three types of physicians: general practitioners, clinical specialists and nursing home physicians. The structure of this table differs from that of the two previous ones. The sum of all horizontal percentages is 100%. Marked differences also appear from this table. In deaths

Tabel 13.8   Cause of death, according to last-mentioned MDEL-action (death certificate study)

	MDEL-action %[3]	No MDEL-action %[3]	Last-mentioned MDEL-action[1]					All actions together n=2361 %	Mortality in The Netherl. 1990[2] n=128786 %
			4a/b n=513 %	4c n=922 %	5 n=244 %	6a/b n=478 %	7 n=204 %		
% last mentioned action	39	61	9	15	4	9	3	39	
Cause of death									
Cancer	59	41	28	53	61	31	68	44	27
Cardiovascular diseases	21	79	17	16	9	21	9	16	30
Diseases of the nervous system (incl. stroke)	43	57	21	9	10	15	2	13	12
Pulmonary diseases	37	63	9	5	8	8	6	7	8
External causes	12	88	1.5	1.1	1.8	1.2	0.3	1.2	4.1
Mental disorders	52	48	2.1	0.7	0.6	1.7	–	1.2	0.9
Other (all other categories)	43	58	21	16	9	23	15	18	18
Total	39	61	100	100	100	100	100	100	100

1) see table 13.7
2) Source: CBS causes-of-death statistics
3) Row percentages

Table 13.9   Type of physician, according to last-mentioned MDEL-action[1]) (death certificate study)

| | Number of questionnaires processed | \multicolumn{5}{c}{Last-mentioned MDEL-action[2])} | MDEL-action | No MDEL-action | Total |
| | | 4a/b | 4c | 5 | 6a/b | 7 | | | |
		%	%	%	%	%	%	%	%
% last mentioned action		9.2	15.0	3.8	8.6	2.7	39.4	60.6	100.0
Type of physician									
General practitioner	2356	6.9	13.4	4.2	5.7	3.7	33.9	66.1	100.0
Specialist	1766	8.7	15.1	3.8	10.0	2.8	40.4	59.6	100.0
Nursing home physician	986	17.3	20.8	3.5	13.9	0.4	55.9	44.1	100.0
Other (=other function and unknown)	89	1.7	1.0	–	0.5	0.6	3.8	96.2	100.0

1)   In contrast to Tables 13.7 and 13.8, Table 13.9 only has row percentages.
2)   See table 13.7.

reported by general practitioners no MDEL-action was performed in 66% of cases. This figure is 60% for specialists, while the percentage for cases reported by nursing home physicians is 44%. The cases in which the nursing home physician performed an MDEL-action are mostly those in which a treatment was withdrawn or withheld.

Also, intensifying alleviation of pain and/or symptoms with the probability taken into account that the end of life would be hastened (question 4c) played a relatively important role. MDEL-actions referred to by question 7 occur very rarely in nursing homes.

The distribution of MDEL-actions for specialists agrees with that found for that in the general population.

This is not the case for general practitioners. The actions related to question 7 are reported relatively more often, i.e. in 3.7% of deaths, while the national average is 2.7%.

13.8 Affirmative answers to question 7

Question 7 is an important part of the standard questionnaire. We repeat the formulation of this question, for the benefit of the reader:

Was the death the consequence of using a drug [*] *prescribed, supplied or administered by you or a colleague* **with the explicit purpose** *of hastening the end of life (or enabling the patient to terminate life himself)?*

Thereafter it was asked who had administered (introduced into the body) the drug. The following categories of answers were possible:

— *patient him/herself in presence of physician*
— *patient him/herself in absence of physician*
— *you or a colleague*
— *a nurse*
— *someone else in presence of physician*
— *someone else in absence of physician*

There were several instances of more than one of these categories being checked. The answers to these questions were ranked as follows:

1. the drug was administered by a physician, regardless of whether others had also administered a drug;
2. the drug was administered by a nurse but not by a physician, regardless of whether others had also administered something;
3. administration by someone other than the patient him/herself, but not (also) by a physician or nurse;
4. administration by patient him/herself, not (also) by a physician, nurse nor someone else.

Table 13.10 Administration of a drug with the explicit purpose of hastening the end of life (death certificate study)

	number n=204	weighted number n=1125	% of total n=41587
Administration (at least also) by physician	151	775	1.9
Administration (also) by nurse (not by physician)	23	193	0.5
Administration by others, not (also) by physician or nurse	9	58	˙0.1
Administration by patient, not (also) by physician, nurse or other	17	82	0.2
Unknown	4	17	0.04
Number of possible cases of euthanasia (see text)	138	701	1.7

[*] One or more drugs may be concerned; morphine is sometimes used for this purpose also.

Table 13.10 shows the distribution of the occurrences over these four categories, both as numbers and as percentages of the national total. Only the first category contains sufficient filled-in questionnaires to permit a reliable estimate to be arrived at for The Netherlands. The distribution of these numbers cannot be interpreted without applying weighting factors (see Appendix E). Therefore, with the greatest possible reservation, the distribution of the weighted numbers for the three other categories are presented.

In principle category 1 contains euthanasia and, if there had not been an explicit request of the patient, acting to terminate life without explicit request. As discussed in Section 11.3 it is clear that not all those who replied by 'yes' to question 7 considered this action as euthanasia. This distinction is of great importance for the interpretation of these results (see Chapter 17).

The action described in category 4 can be considered as assisted suicide. The actions in categories 2 and 3 are, according to the respective definition, also to be considered as euthanasia or as act to terminate life without explicit request. In the definition of euthanasia the physician is not mentioned as 'actor' (definition by Dutch State Committee 1985 [1]). It should be pointed out here that if there had been an act to terminate life by someone else but the patient, physician or nurse, the drug used was prescribed or supplied by a physician. This follows from the formulation of the question.

Figure 13.1 provides detailed information about cases in which the drug was administered by a physician and/or a nurse. The numbers stated in the figure are not weighted. The patient was consulted in most cases. Also in most cases there was an explicit and often also a repeated request. There was an explicit request in 132 cases. These 132 cases are to be considered as the consequence of euthanasia according to the definition by the 'State Committee'. It is also possible that several cases for which questions 5 or 6 of the standard questionnaire were the last ones answered affirmatively could be considered as classifiable as euthanasia. The reason why defining the boundary is sometimes difficult is set out elsewhere in this book (Chapters 3 and 17).

There was a written advance directive of the patient's wishes in half of these cases. There was consultation with a colleague in 126 of the 152 cases.

In the 22 cases in which it was not discussed with the patient the physician felt that discussion was not possible. Five of the 22 deceased had previously expressed their wish for hastening of the end of life. There was an explicit request by relatives or others in 10 of the 22 cases. For 11 of the cases in which such an explicit request had not been made there had been consultations with others, in most instances with several persons (colleague, nursing staff, relatives).

Figure 13.2 provides further information about the 26 cases for which question 7 was answered affirmatively but in which the drug concerned was not administered by the physician and/or nurse.

142

Figure 13.1 Schematic presentation of the number of cases in which a drug was administered by a physician and/or nurse with the explicit purpose of hastening the end of life (numbers not weighted)

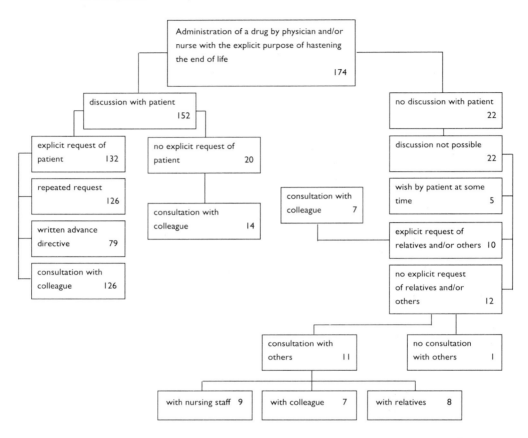

The drug was administered by the patient in 17 cases and this was therefore classified as assisted suicide (category 4). In all cases this happened upon explicit and repeated request of the patient. In 11 cases there was a written statement by the patient and a colleague was consulted in all cases.

It also happened that the drug was administered by someone other than the physician and/or nurse (above mentioned category 3). This occurred in 9 out of 204 cases. There was discussion with the patient in 7 cases while discussion was not possible in 2 cases. In 6 cases the drug was administered upon explicit and repeated request of the patient. These cases are to be classified as euthanasia, as defined by the State Committee.

Figure 13.2 Schematic presentation of the number of cases of assisted suicide and administration of a drug by someone else with the explicit purpose of hastening the end of life (numbers not weighted)

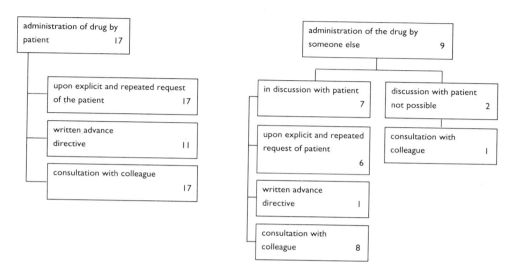

Together with the cases in which administration of the drug was by a physician and/or a nurse one arrives at a weighted number of 701 cases of euthanasia among deaths during the period of August to November 1990 (1.7%).

13.9 Young patients

Requests to terminate life can also occur in the relationship between physicians and minors (up to 18 years of age). There can be two situations; the patients themselves request this or their legal representatives do this.

In principle, a physician is not permitted (except in emergencies) to start or withdraw treatment in a child younger than 16 years of age without permission of their legal representative. In practice, however, the young patient plays a more important role in medical decision-making than the law attributes to him. A child may be very well able to assess its situation and take a well considered decision. This has been taken into account in the Dutch draft law concerning the medical therapy agreement. From the age of 16 years on one can seek therapy from a physician without permission from the legal representative. Furthermore, the draft law considers the maturity of 12- to 16-year-olds. To start or stop a therapy of someone of this age, permission from the child is needed in addition to that of its legal representative.

The study took this into account by establishing three age categories: the group of 0 age (who can never make a request themselves), the group of 1- to 11-year-olds, the older members of which could perhaps request hastening, and the group of 12- to 19-year-olds. Further subdivision, e.g. with age limits of 16 and 18 years was not possible in view of the very small number of deaths in these age groups.

The sample contained only 73 deaths occurring at age 19 years or less. This number was too small to allow generally valid conclusions to be arrived at about MDELs in youngsters. Only a brief description will follow of the findings in some groups.

The sample included 35 deaths in the category 0-age. No MDEL-action was performed in 17 of these cases, while there was an MDEL-action in 18 cases (see Table 13.11).

In two of these cases a drug was administered by the physician with the explicit purpose of hastening the end of life. This action was performed upon explicit request by the parents and after consultation with a colleague.

There were 15 deaths reported for the 1–11 years age group and there was an MDEL-action in 6 of these. These actions varied from actions in which hastening of the end of life had been considered to cases in which hastening the end of life was the explicit purpose.

Of the 23 deaths reported for the age category 12 to 19 years, 19 did not involve an MDEL-action.

One can conclude from these results that actions to terminate life do occur,

Table 13.11 Frequency of last-mentioned MDEL-actions in youngsters (death certificate study)

	Total number in sample	No MDEL-action per-formed	Last-mentioned MDEL-action[1]				
			4a/b	4c	5	6a/b	7
0 year	35	17	3	4	–	9	2
1 – 11 year	15	9	2	1	1	1	1
12 – 19 year	23	19	1	2	–	1	–

1) Taking into account the probability that the end of life was hastened by::
  4a/b withholding or withdrawing a treatment
  4c intensifying alleviation of pain and/or symptoms
In part with the purpose of hastening the end of life by:
  5 intensifying alleviation of pain and/or symptoms.
With the explicit purpose of hastening the end of life by:
  6a/b withholding or withdrawing a treatment ;
  7 prescribing, supplying or administering a drug.

Table 13.12 DNR decisions (death certificate study)

	General practitioner n= 2356 %	Specialist n= 1766 %	Nursing home physician n= 986 %	Total n= 5197 %
Explicitly agreed not to resuscitate[1])	16	60	28	35
– with colleagues	6	48	20	25
– with nursing staff	6	53	23	27
– with patient	8	9	6	8
– with relatives of patient	11	32	18	20
Only implicitly agreed	1	0	36	7
No DNR decision	80	38	33	56
Unknown	3	2	3	2
Total	100	100	100	100

1) The agreement may have been made with one or more of the persons mentioned below.

Table 13.13 Requests to terminate life that were not carried out (death certificate study)

	n= 5197 %
Explicit request that was not carried out [1]):	2.2
– yes, request by patient	1.4
– yes, request by relatives	1.1
– yes, request by others	0.1
No request that was not carried out	92.5
Unknown	5.3
Total	100.0

1) Request could have been made by one or more persons.

there had been an explicit request to terminate life that was not carried out. Two thirds of these requests were made by the patient.

One must obviously be extremely cautious with the interpretation of these data. Nevertheless, the question is a very serious one because it concerns an explicit request. This suggests an important decision situation.

PART IV

PROSPECTIVE STUDY

Participation in the prospective study differed between respondents. As the interviews had taken place during a period of four months, the prospective study started on November 15, 1990 for some respondents, while this date was February 1, 1991 for the last respondents. These last respondents could not participate for the entire period of six months, considering the limited period of time available for the entire study. Data collection was terminated on May 31, 1991. No deaths occurring after this date were included.

14.3 Response, completeness and representativeness

Immediately after the physician interviews 365 (90%) respondents indicated their willingness to participate in the prospective study. Several respondents, particularly specialists, withdrew from this study in the months following, the reason in each case being that filling in the standard questionnaire after each death took too much time. In total, the percentage of respondents participating in the prospective study amounted to 80% of the initial number.

The number of weeks of participation in the prospective study by individual participants was recorded carefully. This information made it possible to derive, for each specialty, weighting factors for the estimation of the number of expected deaths in the prospective study. A summary of these factors is presented in Section E.5. Section C.6 contains a summary of the expected and observed numbers of deaths, listed according to specialty.

The total number of deaths expected was 2220 and the number of questionnaires submitted was 2257, which showed good agreement. Cardiologists reported a few more deaths, nursing home physicians somewhat fewer than expected (see Table C.7). It follows that it can be assumed that physicians participating in the prospective study were, in general, accurate in their reports.

Such completeness does not ensure that the results are representative for all of The Netherlands. To explore this aspect, the distribution according to age, sex and cause of death found in the prospective study was compared with that found for the whole population. In the prospective study, relatively more males were found than had been expected based on the death distribution pattern for the entire country. This could have been a consequence of the coding procedure used in the prospective study. Physicians had possibly occasionally coded a female as male. Another difference was the fraction of cardiovascular diseases. It was somewhat larger in the prospective study than in the national distribution. The distribution according to age and cause of death was virtually identical in all other respects to that found for the whole of The Netherlands (see Table C.8).

The results of the physician interviews made it possible to check whether there was any important difference between those who participated in the prospective study and those who did not do so. There was no significant difference between participants and non-participants with respect to the percentage of respondents indicating that they had, at some time, performed euthanasia or had hastened the end of life without explicit request of the patient.

14.4 Quality of data

The same can be stated about the quality of the prospective study as was stated for that of the death certificate study (Section 12.5). The quality was remarkably good. Most questionnaires were filled in consistently and completely. They contained further information when necessary. This led to adjustments in a small number of cases. In most instances the questionnaires could be used in the condition in which they were received.

The possibility of telephoning respondents (the names of respondents were known to the investigators in this study) to ask them to clarify certain issues was made use of only in a few cases.

Table 15.1   MDEL-actions performed by the physician; comparison of prospective study to death certificate study

	Prospective study		Death certificate study	
	Replies given total n[1])= 2257 %[3])	of which as last mentioned MDEL-action n[1])= 2257 %	Replies given total n[1])= 5197 %[3])	of which as last mentioned MDEL-action n[1])= 5197 %
No MDEL-action performed	**64.6**	**64 .6**	**60.6**	**60.6**
Stratum 0[2])	n.a.	n.a.	9.0	9.0
First contact after the death	2.1	2.1	2.8	2.8
Sudden and totally unexpected death	29.2	29.2	18.1	18.1
Other cases where no MDEL-action was performed (no 'yes' to questions 4 to 7)	33.3	33.3	30.6	30.6
MDEL-action performed	**35.4**	**35.4**	**39.4**	**39.4**
Taking into account the probability that the end of life was hastened by:				
4a withholding a treatment	19.6	5.5	21.6	5.6
4b withdrawing a treatment	13.2	3.5	13.9	3.6
4c intensifying alleviation of pain and/or symptoms	20.2	11.2	25.0	15.0
In part with the purpose of hastening the end of life by:				
5 intensifying alleviation of pain and/or symptoms	7.0	2.6	7.6	3.8
With the explicit purpose of hastening the end of life by:				
6a withholding a treatment	7.2	3.5	7.1	4.3
6b withdrawing a treatment	5.7	4.4	5.1	4.3
7 prescribing, supplying or administering a drug	4.7	4.7	2.7	2.7
Total	**100.0**	**100.0**	**100.0**	**100.0**

1.   Total number of standard questionnaires on which this column is based (plus stratum 0-cases for the death certificate study).

2.   Because no standard questionnaires had been sent of stratum 0 (death certificate study), the distribution over the next three categories is not known. It is known, however, that no MDEL-action was performed in these cases (see section 12.2 and the text of the standard questionnaire). In the death certificate study the 3 categories therefore do not contain stratum 0 deaths.

3.   The percentages in this column add up to more than 100%, because more than one of questions 4 to 7 could be answered with "yes".

hastening the end of life (question 7) occurs more often: 4.7% and 2.7% respectively.

The percentages of deaths in which withholding or withdrawing treatment was stated as last-mentioned MDEL-action (questions 4a and b and 6a and b) agree almost completely: 17.0% and 17.9% in prospective and death certificate studies respectively. The fact that the prospective study yielded fewer reports of intensifying alleviation of pain and/or symptoms in which the probability was taken into account that the end of life would be hastened appears to have two consequences.

The first consequence is that the total percentage of all deaths for which an MDEL-action was performed is lower in the prospective than in the death certificate study. On the other hand, the prospective study showed a higher percentage of deaths for which question 7 was answered in the affirmative. It seems as if respondents of the prospective study were inclined to reply to questions 4 to 7 a little more in extremes. The agreement in the distribution of replies between the two studies is remarkable in all other respects.

15.3 Extent of shortening life

Table F.2 of Appendix F presents in detail the estimated extent of shortening of life for the various 'last-mentioned MDEL-actions'. A first comparison shows that, on the whole, the reported extent of shortening of life was higher in the prospective study than in the death certificate study. The distributions of the extent of shortening of life over the various MDEL-actions, however, are in good agreement. A brief summary follows.

No or only slight shortening of life was reported for a large number of deaths for which one of questions 4a to 4c was the last-mentioned MDEL-action.

In both studies there were about 1% of deaths for which an MDEL-action was performed and for which shortening of life was more than half a year, i.e. in 0.3% of all deaths.

Also, in the prospective study, withholding treatment (question 6a) appears to be as no less serious in terms of shortening of life than the action referred to in question 7.

15.4 Role of the patient in decision-taking

Was it discussed with the patient?

Question 9 of the standard questionnaire concerns discussion with the patient about the 'last-mentioned MDEL-action'. The distribution of replies to this question is shown in Table F.3. It was reported in both studies that no discussion with the patient had taken place in a little more than one half of the deaths for

158

nursing homes (0.4%). The distribution of 'last-mentioned MDEL-actions' according to type of physician shows, in both the prospective and the death certificate studies, that question 7 was answered affirmatively more often by general practitioners (7% and 4%, respectively) and specialists (4% and 3%, respectively) than by nursing home physicians (0.4%).

15.6 Affirmative replies to question 7

Figure 15.1 show a distribution pattern analogous to that in Figure 13.1. The distribution pattern of Figure 15.1 is based on the actual numbers of filled-in standard questionnaires, without weighting. Direct comparison of the numbers in the two figures is therefore not possible. In the prospective study, e.g., there was

Figure 15.1 Schematic presentation of the number of cases in which a drug was administered by a physician and/or nurse with the explicit purpose of hastening the end of life (numbers not weighted)

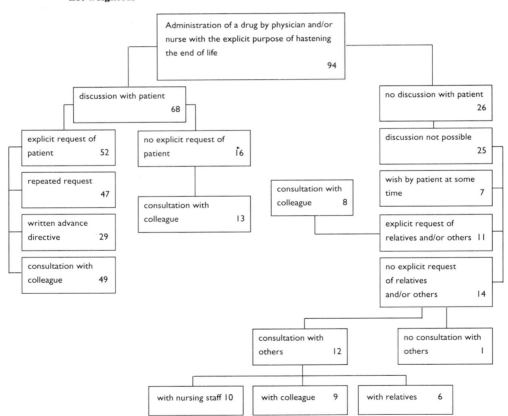

no discussion with the patient in almost one third of all cases (26/94). In the death certificate study this occurred in only one out of 8 patients (22/174). After applying the appropriate weighting to make the figures applicable to the entire Dutch population, it appears from both studies that there was no discussion with the patient in about 20% of cases. For the 26 cases in the prospective study the respondents indicated that no discussion with the patient had been possible in 25 cases. In 7 cases the patient had indicated at some time the wish to have the end of life hastened, while in 11 cases there was an explicit request from relatives and/or others. Consultation with one or more others (colleague, nurse, relatives) occurred in 12 out of 14 cases in which there was no discussion with the patient. There was one case in which the physician consulted no one.

The figure for the prospective study that would be equivalent to Figure 13.2 is not shown here because only 7 and 3 deaths were involved, respectively. There were 7 cases in which the patient himself administered the drug. In all cases this happened after explicit and repeated request of the patient, a written advance directive was available and a colleague was consulted.

15.7 Other findings

Both studies indicate that a decision not to resuscitate (DNR) in cases of possible cardiac or respiratory arrest was explicitly or implicitly taken in advance in somewhat fewer than half the cases (see Table F.11). Based on grouping according to type of physician, general practitioners took such a DNR decision in 17%, specialists in 61% and nursing home physicians in 70% of cases. It is of interest that the prospective and death certificate studies differ with respect to the relationship between explicitly or implicitly deciding on DNR by nursing home physicians. Relatively more cases with implicit decisions were reported in the prospective study. The last question of the standard questionnaire concerned explicit requests to terminate life which were not carried out. This percentage was a little higher in the prospective study than in the death certificate study (3.3% and 2.2%, respectively). Both studies showed that in most cases these were requests by patients which were not carried out.

15.8 The difference between the prospective study and the death certificate study

Size of difference

The similarities and differences between the two studies with respect to distribution of MDEL-actions were discussed in Section 15.2. It was mentioned that respondents in the prospective study apparently were more inclined to choose

elsewhere (see Section 12.5). Within the "in-hospital" and the "elsewhere" groups the response percentages with respect to age, sex and cause of death were again almost constant. Moreover, weighting again corrected the difference between "in-hospital" deaths and "elsewhere" deaths.

The data of the prospective study were obtained from a limited number of known responders. Of these, 20% did not participate in the prospective study but did participate in the physician interview study. The period during which participating respondents took part in the prospective study is known exactly. It can be assumed that they provided virtually complete information. There may be a slightly greater risk of bias in the data obtained from clinical specialists, while general practitioners probably supplied very complete information. However, the greatest difference between the answers to question 7 was found in the general practitioners' group.

The questionnaires used in both studies were identical from question 4 onwards. However, it was discovered later that there was a slight *difference between the questionnaires*, in a footnote to question 7. In the death certificate study the wording of the footnote was: "morphine is sometimes used for this purpose also". In the prospective study this footnote was formulated: "morphine can be prescribed for this purpose also". It cannot be excluded that the latter formulation led the respondent to reply in the affirmative to question 7, while in fact morphine was used to intensify alleviation of pain and/or symptoms.

The death certificate study relates to deaths during the period of August to November 1990. The prospective study covered deaths in the period of 15 November 1990 to 1 June 1991. Theoretically, it is conceivable that *seasonal fluctuations* might have caused the observed differences in the incidence of euthanasia, although this is not very likely.

Respondent-related explanations

The position of the respondent, changes in behaviour, reporting procedure, differences in interpretation and learning effects will be discussed briefly.

The *position of the respondent* can be of importance in the clinical situation. An estimate would be that in the death certificate study about one half of the questionnaires were filled in by physicians in training. This also occurred in the prospective study, but far less frequently. It is conceivable that a physician in training would be more reticent when filling in the questionnaire than would a clinical specialist. However, this difference could not have been a factor for deaths that had occurred at the deceased's home; considerable differences were also found for this category.

Theoretically it is conceivable that after the interview participants in the prospective study *changed their behaviour* with respect to MDELs by more often performing actions described by question 7.

Another factor that could have been of importance when filling in the questionnaire is the *reporting procedure* for euthanasia that applied as of 1 November 1990. It is definite that willingness of physicians to report euthanasia has increased since the new reporting procedure was introduced. It cannot be excluded that this change influenced the replies in the questionnaire in a number of cases. Most deaths in the death certificate study occurred before November 1, 1990, while all deaths in the prospective study occurred thereafter.

It is not inconceivable that there were differences in *interpretation* between the respondents of the two studies. The respondents in the death certificate study had no information other than the questionnaire and the accompanying letter. All respondents in the prospective study had participated in the physician interviews and, therefore, had discussed one or more cases out of their own practice in detail with a trained interviewer for two and a half hours. All concepts of crucial importance which occurred in the standard questionnaire were discussed repeatedly on this occasion. Considering the smaller percentage of affirmative answers to questions 4c and 5 and the greater percentage of affirmative answers to question 7 it is conceivable that participants in the prospective study were more inclined to report that administering morphine and similar drugs was done with the explicit purpose of hastening the end of life. Occasional enquiries with respondents confirmed this conjecture. A respondent without the experience of an earlier interview may in good faith describe a certain action as belonging to questions 4c or 5. However, with the experience of the earlier interview he may well assign a more serious intention to the same action and thereore classify it as 'affirmative' in question 7. This possible explanation is supported by the comment of a great number of respondents that the interview had clarified their thinking about MDELs.

Finally there is the possibility of a learning-effect. Participants in the prospective study often filled in a relatively large number of questionnaires (an average of seven questionnaires each) while this activity was much more spread out over participants in the death certificate study. Familiarity with the questionnaire may have led the respondent to reply negatively to questions 4 to 6, knowing that question 7 was still to come.

Considering these possible explanations for the differences found between the answers to questions 4c, 5 and 7, the investigators are inclined to consider as most important the fact that respondents in the prospective study changed their approach with respect to their intention when administering morphine due to their recent intensive confrontation with thinking about this complex of problems. Chance variations probably also contribute to the differences found.

The results of the study as to the interpretation of questions 4 to 7, described in Section 11.3, also play a role in this conclusion. The study just mentioned showed that in a number of cases respondents replied in the affirmative to question 7 in instances which they themselves would not have considered as euthanasia. There is clearly a gradual transition between the intentions described in questions 4c, 5 and 7, at least as far as morphine and comparable drugs are concerned. This can have caused physicians who participated in the interviews to state more easily that they had in mind the explicit purpose of hastening the end of life when intensifying alleviation of pain and/or symptoms. This again agrees with the fact that the percentage of euthanasia in the total number of deaths was estimated to be lower in the physician interviews than in the prospective study.

The significance of the above considerations for the definitive estimate of the incidence of euthanasia and other MDELs will be discussed in Chapter 17.

PART V

INTEGRATION

16. Additional interviews

16.1 Introduction

The sample of physicians was designed to obtain information that, in principle, would cover about 95% of all deaths in The Netherlands. These 95% are not fully representative of all deaths because in the remaining 5% various deaths occur which have special characteristics. However, these groups are so small that it is not possible to obtain information from a reasonably sized random sample of physicians.

Special groups for which no or insufficient information could be collected via the physician sample and which are briefly discussed in this chapter are:

- newborn babies;
- older children;
- psychiatric patients;
- AIDS patients.

The first three groups present the problem that they are not (yet) able to take a decision. The last two groups are characterised by a very specific type of suffering.

Four special studies would have been required to collect data in a manner that would be comparable to that used for the other deaths. This could not be done within the period of time available. The Commission and the investigators, however, considered it of importance to get an impression of the decision-making processes in these special groups in comparison to the findings for the group representing 95% of all deaths. A qualitative description of the decision-making process in these groups and of the level of development of opinions in this particular sector of health care are presented.

To achieve this, informants were consulted about who were considered experts in the particular sector of health care. Twelve experts were interviewed in total. The interviews lasted from 1½ to 3 hours. During these interviews several questions were asked which were specific for the particular group, in addition to questions taken from the questionnaire of the physician interviews. All respondents were interviewed by the authors.

16.2 Newborns

During 1990 a total of 1399 0-year olds died in The Netherlands, more than half of this number during the first week of life. The medical possibilities for keeping premature babies and severely handicapped newborns alive have increased greatly in the past ten to fifteen years. Physicians therefore increasingly have to face questions as to whether to start or continue a particular treatment for a particular newborn. The situation thus arising and requiring a decision differs from other situations discussed in this report in several characteristics:

– It is often not possible to immediately make a clear diagnosis regarding chances of survival, risk of permanent damage to health and chances of an existence which will permit at least a minimal chance of human communication; this often requires at least one or more days of observation. This means that treatment has to be started in almost all premature babies or newborns. When further prolongation of life in fact only means prolongation of suffering or if prognosis for (the quality of) later life is very poor, a decision has to be taken (in second instance) about withdrawing treatment.
– The patient cannot in any way participate in the decision-making process. The opinion of parents, which can vary widely for comparable patients, is of great importance in the process of arriving at a decision.

There are ten centres in The Netherlands where most (very) premature babies and newborns with serious abnormalities are treated. Situations in which an important decision concerning the end of life of a newborn has to be taken occur fairly frequently in these centres. This makes the forming of an opinion about MDELs within this group of specialists more important than if one were confronted with such a situation only incidentally.

Much has been published in the international literature about medical decision-making with respect to newborns. In The Netherlands, the Health Council published a report in 1975 [10], also both the Dutch Paediatric Society and the Royal Dutch Medical Association have published reports [11,12]. This means that the shaping of public opinion regarding this particular area, within and beyond the professional groups, is considerably more advanced than regarding the other three groups to be discussed in this chapter. The medical profession generally feels that not everything that can possibly be done should be done.

Something can be reported about the number and the type of decisions in this area. Some important MDEL was taken in certainly half of all deaths in neonatology centres. Data from the death certificate study are in agreement here (see Section 13.9). A quantitative study of MDELs is in progress in several neonatology centres. It was stated above that this kind of situation requiring a decision often arises because a prognosis cannot be made with certainty immediately after birth and treatment is therefore started. By far most important MDELs in neonatology concern withdrawing or withholding treatment. When withdrawing treatment, artificial respiration in particular, it can be desirable to increase the dose of sedating drugs in order not to prolong needlessly the suffering of the dying newborn. It is very exceptional that an act to terminate life is performed in a newborn who would probably remain alive without medical support.

A special situation requiring a decision arises because there are increasing possibilities of surgical interventions for children with very serious congenital abnormalities. In such situations, surgery can lead to a considerably increased life expectancy. The question as to the quality of life can be a very important one in the considerations of parents and physicians, if life has to be maintained in this manner. Difficult situations can also arise if surgery can only partially correct certain abnormalities which are not immediately life-threatening. In such a case and considering present-day medical possibilities the newborn may only have a life perspective of very serious invalidity. In such a situation sometimes the decision is taken to terminate life after extensive consultations with other physicians and the parents. Points of view with respect to these problems differ within the pediatric profession.

The (expected) quality of life plays an important role in the decisions concerning newborns that were discussed here. It is currently under discussion whether several groups could be distinguished: some where treatment can always be withdrawn, some where this must never occur and a "grey area" between the two.

The experts who were consulted felt that the kinds of decisions discussed above could best be left to parents and physicians. Nursing staff often have an important voice in the preparatory decision process. However, the physician has the final responsibility. In most instances parents and physicians seem to agree with each other. If this is not the case, treatment usuallycontinues. The decision that has been taken should be tested, but only afterwards and not primarily by a judge.

The persons who were interviewed indicated that the quality of the decision-taking in this field has improved considerably in recent years because of the development of opinions within the pediatric profession.

16.3 Older children

In 1990, 541 children 1 to 11 years of age and 556 children 12 to 19 years of age died in The Netherlands. The decision situation with respect to older children has the following characteristics:

- As the child gets older it has more to say with respect to treatment, withdrawing treatment and, possibly also hastening the end of life. This was discussed in Section 13.9.
- In all cases parents or guardians have an important voice. There can be differences in opinion between child and parents about the continuation of treatment.

– Contrary to the treatment of newborns, the treatment of older ill children is spread over a large number of hospitals. The individual pediatrician is confronted relatively infrequently with MDELs. Such situations occur relatively more often only in a few specialised centres, e.g. in pediatric oncology. Most children suffering from cancer eventually die at home. This means that the final decision is often taken without participation of the pediatrician, while this remains an extremely rare situation for the general practitioner.

The lack of information in the literature and the limited number of interviews that could be held in the context of this investigation only allow very general statements to be made.

The fact that MDELs in pediatrics, with the exception of neonatology, are not made in a defined and limited number of centres probably contributed to the fact that public opinion concerning these matters is little developed.

It is certain that MDELs are sometimes made for older children also. Most likely, a smaller number of deaths is involved here than is the case for newborns. This is confirmed by the results of Section 13.9. An important reason for this situation is that many deaths in older children are the consequence of accidents, situations in which few MDELs are taken. In children, this kind of decision will mostly be of importance in the final stage of an incurable disease. As many seriously ill children eventually die at home, collaboration between specialist and general practitioner is most important. Both should be involved when a decision has to be taken. Both general practitioners and specialists should also be involved in further opinion-forming and in the development of procedures.

16.4 Psychiatry

In 1990, the number of deaths in psychiatric institutions in The Netherlands was at least 1267. Many of these were older psychiatric patients admitted permanently who suffer from an incurable somatic disease. The MDELs arising do not differ in essence from those described earlier in this report. In a relatively great number of cases patients will not be able to take a decision.

A situation that differs from those discussed previously is the one in which a request for assisted suicide is made by a patient who does not suffer from a serious somatic disease. Such requests are made relatively frequently by persons suffering from a severe psychiatric disorderand a psychiatrist is asked to give his opinion or even arrive at a decision about such a request. Important characteristics of this situation are:

– There is an explicit request by a patient. It is extraordinarily difficult to answer the question as to whether this patient is able to assess his situation and to take a decision adequately.

– Often patients are involved who do not suffer from a life-threatening disease and who, in principle could go on living for many years. In this respect the request for assisted suicide differs from that of a patient suffering from an incurable, somatic disease.

A request for assisted suicide made by a person not suffering from a serious somatic disease does not always need to have a psychiatric component. The number of requests for assisted suicide by persons who after careful deliberation have decided that they do not wish to continue their existence may even be greater. However, the additional interviews were limited to the area of psychiatry.

There have been several committees in recent years that were involved with the subject of assisted suicide. In 1985 the "State committee on euthanasia" wrote in its advice: "The State committee is of the opinion that its proposals related to unpunished assistance with suicide must be limited to the situation in which, according to the committee's opinion, assisted suicide is admissible. The committee does not at this point consider it justified to make proposals related to abolishing punishability of assistance with suicide beyond the cases indicated for termination of life upon request without punishment, *as the issues involved have not yet been clarified sufficiently by scientific and social opinion-forming*" [1].

The "Suicide" committee of the Health Council of The Netherlands wrote in its advice: "The commission has decided not to produce an exhaustive discussion about the problem of assisted suicide; the relevant chapter is *not meant to be more than a contribution to continuing social discussion. Moreover it did not succeed in producing a unanimous opinion about this problem*" [13].

Both committees indicate that public opinion concerning assisted suicide has not yet been sufficiently developed. The experts interviewed agree.

In the recently published report of the Dutch Association for Voluntary Euthanasia, the "Assistance with problems related to suicide" committee feels that public discussion has made further advances. It writes: "Our committee feels that with respect to shaping of public opinion it can be assumed that most of those who are not religiously oriented consider assisted suicide acceptable under certain conditions and that most of those who are religiously oriented reject the idea of assisted suicide" [14].

It is difficult to assess a request for assisted suicide and it may, in some ways, even be impossible. When a patient suffering from a serious permanent depression makes such a request, it can be considered as a symptom of the disease implying restricted ability to arrive at a judgement, but it can also be the result of a balanced judgement by a patient who decides that he can no longer bear severe psychic suffering. The problem of an uncertain prognosis for such conditions is important. There are examples of patients who have lived what is for them a very satisfactory life after their very serious and repeated requests for assisted suicide had been refused.

The experts interviewed feel that in psychiatry one is extremely reticent with assisting in suicide. Requests for assisted suicide are not infrequent, while persistence with such a requestis infrequent. The number of cases of assistance with suicide on the basis of exclusively psychiatric suffering can be estimated to be probably less than 10 annually in The Netherlands.

The above indicates that taking a decision with respect to assisted suicide because of exclusively psychiatric suffering is extremely difficult. Uncertainty about the significance of the request and about diagnosis and prognosis requires not only extreme caution but moreover very special expertise. Therefore it is not surprising that public opinion-forming progresses only very slowly. The conclusions to be drawn later in this book do explicity not refer to this area.

16.5 AIDS patients

The diagnosis of AIDS had been made at least 1800 times in The Netherlands up to mid-1991. It can be assumed that, over the years, about half of these patients died. Patients in the terminal stage of AIDS are almost always under treatment by a general practitioner, an internist or both. Thus they belong to the group of deaths investigated in the three part-studies. The diagnosis of AIDS also occurred in several cases that were discussed in the physician interviews. The total number, however, was not sufficiently large to be reported on separately. The reason for a brief discussion in this section is that this group has at least two important characteristics:

– a variable but nevertheless very predictable course of illness, more so than, e.g., in most forms of cancer;
– most patients belong to a relatively well defined group of young men who are well informed about the course of their disease and know what they can expect.

MDELs are often taken in this group of patients. Often it has to be decided whether to withdraw or to withhold treatment. Moreover, probably more than half of all AIDS patients raise the issue of euthanasia or assisted suicide. According to a global estimate 10 to 20% of all AIDS patients die due to euthanasia or assisted suicide. This agrees with the results of the only study that contains relevant data [15]. This latter, not representative, study among the relatives of 52 AIDS deaths, showed that euthanasia was performed in 13 cases.

The fact that euthanasia and assisted suicide were not rare in this group of patients is in agreement with the results of the three part-studies. Euthanasia was requested more often by relatively young men with a serious terminal disease. Also performance of euthanasia and assisted suicide occurred more often in this group.

17. Medical decisions concerning the end of life (MDELs): Estimates

17.1 Introduction

The results of the three part-studies are considered together in this chapter. Attention is particularly directed to the estimates that can be arrived at on the basis of these studies. Several other characteristics of the decisions and actions investigated are also discussed. The description of the background of decisions and of other important aspects is not repeated here. These were discussed on the basis of the interview results in Chapters 6 to 8 and comparisons between the death certificate study and the prospective study were made in Chapter 15.

Table 17.1 presents important data concerning the estimates. This table is intended as support for the reader and can only be interpreted properly if the present chapter is read. The table presents estimates and the confidence intervals indicating the accuracy of these estimates. On the basis of all available information and taking into account various advantages and disadvantages of the individual (part) studies the opinion of the investigators as to what represents an acceptable estimate is always indicated. This estimate, considered reasonable by the investigators, is always stated as one percentage or one number for the sake of clarity. The reader should keep in mind that these estimates only try to approach the actual situation as well as possible. In situations where differences occur between the death certificate study and the prospective study, more weight is generally attached to results of the death certificate study because of the greater number of deaths and the method of sampling.

One should also keep in mind that there sometimes are gradual transitions between the various types of Medical Decisions concerning the End of Life. This too should be considered in the interpretation of the estimates. These boundary areas will be discussed first.

17.2 Boundary areas

The entire area of MDELs is classified according to four important questions (Chapter 3):

1. What did the physician do?
2. What was the physican's intention in doing this?
3. Did the patient request this intervention?
4. Was the patient able (or not) to indicate his or her opinion about this intervention?

Each MDEL could be classified into a particular category if each of these four questions was answered clearly. If, e.g., a physician administered a drug with the explicit purpose of hastening the end of life and the patient had requested this action, this complies with the definition of euthanasia as used in The Netherlands. This action will then be discussed in the interview by means of the series of questions regarding euthanasia. The above mentioned four questions also served as the basic structure for the standard questionnaire used for the death certificate study and the prospective study.

The combined information from the part-studies confirms that the total extent of MDELs can be assessed adequately provided one accepts that categorisation can never be absolute. The boundary areas arising from the above mentioned questions will now be discussed briefly, together with two other classification problems.

Question 1: What did the physician do? A physician can perform one or more actions (withdrawing or withholding treatment, administer or prescribe drugs). This does not give rise to confusion. Confusion can arise, however, if more than one actor is involved in the action. If a patient terminates life with a drug prescribed by the physician this is assisted suicide. If first the patient and the physician thereafter administer something, we classify this in this investigation as euthanasia although the termination of life possibly started as assisted suicide. Then there are situations in which the patient together with others administers the drug prescribed by the physician. It then becomes difficult to decide whether this is euthanasia or assisted suicide. Although strictly speaking the distinction between euthanasia and assisted suicide only depends on the identity of the person who administers the drug, in medical practice this difference appears to be more important in certain cases than in others. For a terminal patient who has at most a few hours or days of life left, the decision as to who administers the drug is less weighty than that in the case of a patient with a serious illness whose life can last several more months in relatively good physical condition. For many physicians there is a much greater difference in the latter situation between who administers the drug than in the former.

Question 2: The intention of the physician. The purpose of medicine is the alleviation of pain and symptoms once cure is no longer possible. In the terminal stage of a disease it can be necessary to intensify the alleviation of pain and/or symptoms to the extent that the physician must consider the probability that this may hasten the end of life. On the other hand there may be situations in which hastening of the end of life may be the explicit purpose of the physician (obviously also derived from the aim to terminate suffering). If a physician uses muscle relaxants without artificial respiration the aim can be nothing but hastening of the end of life: the patient will stop breathing. The physician may not always be able to define his intention precisely if he uses morphine in situations in which the life of terminal patients will be shortened by only a few hours or days, if at all.

Questions 3 and 4: The request and the (full) ability of the patient to take a decision. The situation is clear for most decisions. A patient, e.g., has made an explicit request or a patient is totally unable to take a decision because he is unconscious. However, there also are situations in which the patient shows some ability to express his wishes while this expression cannot be considered an explicit request. It is also possible that a patient made a request to terminate life at some time in the past but that his condition deteriorated so quickly that it was no longer possible to make an explicit request during the last weeks of life. In some patients and in some situations it can be difficult to make a clear distinction between the ability and inability to take a decision.

Shortening of life. In nearly all cases physicians were prepared to give an estimate of the amount of time by which the life of a patient was shortened due to a particular action. The uncertainty that surrounds such estimates (see Section 3.5) should always be considered also. It might perhaps be better, however, to think in terms of not prolonging life rather than of shortening of life, particularly in connection with withholding or withdrawing treatment. Physicians sometimes stated that they had decided to no longer prolong suffering or not to extend senselessly the process of dying and that, in their opinion, the term "shortening of life" really did not apply.

Euthanasia. It is often stated explicitly that withdrawing or withholding treatment upon explicit request of the patient should not be considered as euthanasia according to thedefinition applied in The Netherlands. Nevertheless some people feel that e.g. ceasing artificial respiration upon request of the patient, leading to the end of life within a very short period of time, should be considered as euthanasia.

The examples presented above show that producing an estimate of the number of cases of euthanasia and of the purposeful termination of life by action or omission without request, is only justified if information is also collected about these boundary areas.

17.3 Euthanasia and assisted suicide

Numbers and percentages

Whenever possible, estimates are presented as percentages of the total annual number of deaths. The reason is that the total number of deaths differs from year to year. Because absolute numbers are often mentioned in the discussion about euthanasia and other MDELs, the percentages concerned were translated into absolute numbers for the year 1990.

Some of the MDELs discussed do not relate to deceased patients only. Estimates related to such decisions are presented only in absolute numbers. Relevant results of comparable investigations will also be discussed.

Euthanasia

The three part-studies show that euthanasia was performed in 1.7% of all deaths (death certificate study, Table 13.10), 1.9% (physician interviews) or 2.6% (prospective study, Table F.10). The difference between the estimates based on the death certificate study and on the prospective study is probably due to the existence of a boundary area between euthanasia and intensifying of the alleviation of pain and/or symptoms. This was discussed in detail in Chapter 15. In the prospective study more of this boundary area probably was included in the estimate of euthanasia and of performing a life terminating act without the patient's explicit request. In the physician interviews cases are discussed which in the respondent's opinion can be considered cases of euthanasia. Here there is a slight chance of an overestimate due to counting cases twice while in the death certificate study there is a slight chance of an underestimate because of the problem of distinction between euthanasia and the alleviation of pain and/or symptoms. Based on the three part-studies it can be assumed that euthanasia occurs in about 1.8% of all deaths. All three studies suggest that euthanasia was performed by general practitioners in two thirds of these cases. In terms of absolute numbers this means that in the year 1990 about 2300 cases of euthanasia occurred and that euthanasia was carried out by general practitioners in 1550 of these cases (2.9% of all deaths for general practitioners). The specialists performed euthanasia in the remaining cases (1.4% of deaths for specialists), with the exception of some 20 cases where it was performed by nursing home physicians.

Comparable results were obtained in two other recently published studies. The first study involved a postal survey among general practitioners [16]. In this study a description of euthanasia was given first, then it was asked if and how often the general practitioner had performed euthanasia and assisted suicide (according to the definition given). Based on these results the author estimated that in recent years in The Netherlands euthanasia or assisted suicide was performed an average of 2000 times a year. If we add the corresponding estimates from our investigation (see later on in this section) we arrive at about 1900 cases when euthanasia or assisted suicide were performed annually by general practitioners.

A study among nursing home physicians in which a questionnaire was used that was almost identical to the one used for general practitioners mentioned above led to the conclusion that in recent years nursing home physicians performed euthanasia ten times per year in The Netherlands [17]. This order of magnitude agrees completely with that found by us. It is obvious that euthanasia in a nursing home is very rare.

Earlier, mainly foreign, reports mention a number of cases of euthanasia in

The Netherlands far greater than the 2300 reported here. The numbers vary from 5000 to 8000 cases [18-20] to 20 000 [21,22].

Two thirds of the euthanasia cases concern cancer patients. Schudel and Bartelds also reached this conclusion in their study [23,24]. The number of cases of euthanasia in the oldest age group (80+) was less than could have been expected on the basis of the mortality distribution in The Netherlands, but was greater in the age groups up to 65. Most cases were seriously ill patients with only a brief life expectancy. The findings of Van der Wal [25,26] are comparable to these results.

Assisted suicide

Assisted suicide occurs in 0.2% (death certificate study), 0.3% (physician interviews) or 0.4% (prospective study) of all deaths, according to the results of the three part-studies. If 0.3% is taken as a reasonable estimate, this would be equivalent to almost 400 cases in 1990. The general practitioner assisted in almost all cases. However, the comment must be made that in this estimate, cases in which the patient first took some drug and the physician subsequently administered a drug are considered as euthanasia, regardless of whether the initial intention of the physician had been to administer a drug also. The reliability of this estimate is somewhat less than that for the number of cases of euthanasia, because of the definition problem as well as because of the much smaller number of cases involved.

Requests for euthanasia and assisted suicide

In the physician interviews requests for euthanasia were discussed in three ways, depending on the period of time involved:

— requests for euthanasia or assisted suicide in due course;
— requests for euthanasia or assisted suicide in the foreseeable future;
— explicit requests for euthanasia or assisted suicide which were not acceded to by the physician.

The first question was concerned with a request to perform euthanasia or assisted suicide in due course, when suffering would have become unbearable. In total, some 25 000 requests of this nature are made to physicians in The Netherlands. General practitioners receive almost 16 000, and nursing home physicians about 450 requests annually.

Furthermore, there was the question as to requests for euthanasia or assisted suicide in the foreseeable future. Such requests are made some 9000 times to physicians in The Netherlands; of these more than 5000 are made to general practitioners. This means that a general practitioner usually receives such a request a little less than once annually. Obviously the frequency of such requests is distributed unevenly, depending on e.g. the structure of the practice and the physician's views on euthanasia.

This estimate is consistent with earlier ones. Van der Wal [16] arrived at 5000 requests made annually to general practitioners for euthanasia or assisted suicide. The Dutch Institute for Primary Health Care (NIVEL) calculated that the general practitioner receives 1.0 to 2.3 requests per 4 years [24]. Oliemans found in a 1985 study of 25 general practitioners in The Hague 2 requests per 3 years per general practitioner [27]. A subsequent study the year therafter yielded one request per two years [23]. All these data are in good agreement with those of the present study. A 1986 study among general practitioners in Amsterdam produced higher numbers, i.e. an average of three requests per general practitioner per year [28].

The number of requests made to nursing home physicians concerning the foreseeable future was 225. Van der Wal [17] found an identical number for nursing home physicans.

The number of requests for euthanasia is considerably larger than the number of times euthanasia is carried out. Obviously, some of the requests are not acceded to. Most of the times this was because there were alternatives for the patient or the request, in the opinion of the physician, had not been properly and duly considered. In some cases euthanasia will no longer be necessary because the patient dies before suffering becomes unbearable.

In each of the three part-studies a question was asked as to explicit requests for euthanasia that had not been acceded to. In 1.4% (death certificate study) to 2.5% (prospective study) an explicit request of the patient for euthanasia or assisted suicide was not actually carried out prior to the death of the patient. This would mean that, annually, 2000 to 3000 explicit requests for euthanasia or assisted suicide are not acceded to.

During the physician interviews a question was asked as to explicit requests for euthanasia which were not acceded to, also including requests by patients who had not yet died. Together, the answers yielded an estimate of 4000 explicit but not acceded to requests for euthanasia or assisted suicide annually. One could conclude from this difference that euthanasia or assisted suicide were refused to a number of patients who had not died shortly thereafter. At least some of these cases were persons suffering from mental illness. Physical suffering also can appear unbearable and hopeless for some time while the situation then improves considerably (in some cases of cancer chemotherapy, e.g.).

If we add the numbers of cases of euthanasia, assisted suicide and not acceded-to explicit requests, there still remains a difference of more than 2000 cases when this total is compared to the estimated number of requests in the foreseeable future for euthanasia and assisted suicide. Not considering the variability of the individual estimates, a possible explanation for this difference can be that not each request for euthanasia or assisted suicide in the foreseeable future was seen by the physician as an explicit request. Also, a physician can, in a certain way, prevent an explicit request from arising if he is not prepared to accede to such a request for euthanasia or assisted suicide. Moreover, a number of patients may have died before the request was acceded to.

More than half the number of requests refused originated from men; the oldest age group was relatively less represented.

17.4 Other MDELs

Performing a life-terminating act without explicit request of the patient

It is possible to make an estimate, based on the data of the death certificate and prospective studies, of the number of cases in which the physician prescribes, supplies or administers a drug with the explicit purpose of hastening the end of life while the patient has not made an explicit request. According to the death certificate study this occurred in 0.8%, and accordingto the prospective study in 1.6%, of all deaths. Both studies suggest that there was discussion with the patient in some 40% of cases but there had not been an explicit request. In all cases where the decision had not been discussed, this would simply not have been possible, except in one case in the prospective study. In about one quarter of the studies in which discussion was not possible the patient had at some time expressed the wish to have life terminated.

In situations in which there was no discussion with the patient and this was not possible, there always had been consultation with one or more others (relatives, colleagues), except in one case in each of the two studies.

The estimated shortening of life for cases without explicit request was less in the prospective than in the death certificate study (less than one week in 75% and 38% of cases, respectively). The distribution in the prospective study agrees well with that found from the physician interviews (Chapter 6). Therefore one can assume that in the prospective study also the boundary area between the alleviation of pain and/or symptoms on the one hand and performing a life-terminating act on the other is largely included in the latter group, all the more because the same respondents were involved. This also agrees with the conclusion of Section 15.8 in which the difference between affirmative replies to question 7 in the death certificate study and in the prospective study is discussed.

The estimated shortening of life found in the death certificate study was more than 6 months in two cases. Such cases were not found in the prospective study.

One can estimate that, based on the death certificate and prospective studies in 0.8% to 1.6% of deaths a physician prescribed, supplied or administered a drug with the explicit purpose of hastening the end of life without explicit request of the patient. If one limits this estimate to patients with whom it was not discussed and who never had indicated the wish to have the end of life hastened, one arrives at the percentages of 0.3% and 0.7% respectively. The first of the two estimates is more likely to apply than the second one, as was already pointed out several times previously. The two first values are therefore considered as best estimates. Almost all cases concern patients with whom discussion was no longer possible and whose life was only slightly shortened by this act.

Extensive questions as to performing a life-terminating act without the patients request were asked in the physician interviews. Chapter 6 states that not all respondents interpreted these questions in the same way. Therefore a clear distinction cannot be made between these acts and the alleviation of pain and/or symptoms that possibly may also have hastened the end of life. It is not well possible to make an estimate of the number of cases in which life-terminating acts were performed without explicit request of the patient based on the physician interviews (see Section 6.9). Of the 97 cases discussed in the interviews there were 2 in which discussion with the patient would have been possible but did not occur, while the patient also had not indicated anything about terminating life. Furthermore, among the 64 cases in which discussing with the patient neither had been possible nor had there been any indication of the patient's wishes, there were five cases in which the physician had not consulted anyone else. Finally there was one case in the interview study in which discussion with the patient was not possible and the shortening of life was of more than six months. This patient apparently was, in the opinion of his physician, not in the terminal phase of his illness.

If the information obtained in the three part-studies is combined, the following conclusions can be drawn:

1. On an annual basis there are, in The Netherlands, some thousand cases (0.8% of all deaths) for which physicians prescribe, supply or administer a drug with the explicit purpose of hastening the end of life without an explicit request of the patient.
2. In more than half of these cases the decision was discussed with the patient or the patient had previously indicated his wish for hastening the end of life. In several hundred cases there was no discussion with the patient and there also was no known wish from the patient for hastening the end of life.
3. In virtually all cases seriously ill and terminal patients were involved who obviously were suffering a great deal and no longer were able to express their wishes.
4. In several cases no consultation with others (relatives, colleagues) took place.
5. There was a small number of cases in which the decision might have been discussed with the patient.

6. Also in a small number of cases life was shortened by more than half a year. Apparently these patients were not in the terminal phase of their illness.

The alleviation of pain and/or symptoms

A question about the use of the alleviation of pain and/or symptoms was asked in each of the three part-studies, particularly as to the use of morphine or morphine-like drugs in doses that could possibly shorten life. Estimates, as percentages of total deaths, are 16.3% (physician interviews), 18.8% (death certificate study) and 13.8% (prospective study), respectively. The first two estimates are probably closer to reality than that based on the prospective study. It is reasonable to assume the figure of 17.5% of all deaths in which the alleviation of pain and/or symptoms was the most important MDEL-action if one wishes to limit oneself to the use of one value only. The figure of 17.5% of all deaths for the year 1990 amounts to 22 500 cases. Part of the difference between the estimates of the first two studies and the prospective one can probably be explained by shifts in the boundary area between euthanasia and acting to hasten the end of life without explicit request of the patient on the one hand and the alleviation of pain and/or symptoms on the other hand. This boundary area was mostly classified as euthanasia and acting to hasten the end of life without explicit request in the prospective study, while in the other two studies it was grouped under alleviation of pain and/or symptoms (see Section 15.8).

The difference between the percentages of affirmative replies to question 7 between the death certificate study (2.7%) and the prospective study (4.7%) could be considered, with the necessary reservations, as an indication of the size of this boundary area. This implies that in about 2% of all deaths one cannot distinguish clearly whether euthanasia or acts to hasten the end of life were involved, or intensification of the alleviation of pain and/or symptoms with, at least in part, the purpose of hastening the end of life. This estimate is also consistent with the results of the physician interviews for which this boundary area was obtained from the data presented in Chapters 6 and 7. This 2% fraction is included in the above mentioned figure of 17.5%.

In 65% (physician interviews) to 80% (death certificate and prospective studies) of all cases the physician intensified the alleviation of pain and/or symptoms and took into account the probability that the end of life would be hastened. In 20% to 30% (physician interviews) the physicians indicated that hastening the end of life was also partly the purpose. In the interviews physicians indicated that, in 6% of the cases, hastening the end of life was the explicit purpose. These cases again confirm the existence of a boundary area between euthanasia and the alleviation of pain and/or symptoms. The general practitioner was the treating physician in about one third of the cases, the specialist in 40% to 50% of cases and the nursing home physician in the remaining cases.

The three part-studies show that for most patients the shortening of life involved at most a few hours or days. In the death certificate and the prospective studies physicians estimated that in about one third of all cases there was no shortening of life whatsoever. Cancer was the most important diagnosis in more than half of all cases in which the alleviation of pain and/or symptoms was intensified. The patients were relatively young compared to the age distribution of all deaths in The Netherlands. This holds particularly if hastening the end of life was partly the purpose.

Withdrawing and withholding treatment in the death certificate and prospective studies

In the death certificate and prospective studies a question was asked as to withholding or withdrawing treatment. The distribution of these replies is shown in Table 17.1. Withdrawing or withholding treatment occurs as last-mentioned MDEL-action in 17.9% (death certificate study) and 17.0% (prospective study) of all deaths. A reasonable estimate is 17.5% of all deaths, which amounts to some 22 500 cases in 1990. In slightly more than half the cases the physician took into account the probability that the end of life would be hastened. In the other cases hastening of the end of life was the explicit purpose. The decision to withhold treatment in particular had important consequences in terms of shortening of life in some cases.

There are no comparable data in the literature that suggest the percentages of deaths of patients for whom treatment was withdrawn or withheld. However, there are studies concerning special groups of patients. Neu discusses the deaths in a hospital dialysis department in the United States for the years between 1966 and 1983. Out of 704 patients deceased, 155 died because dialysis was withdrawn (22%). This was done upon request for 66 (9%) patients [29]. This latter percentage is consistent with that found in a Dutch study of dialysis patients: 8% of the deaths occurred because of voluntarily withdrawn dialysis [30]. Dialysis patients, however, are not considered to be a group that could be seen as representative for all deaths. They will behave differently in a several respects because they depend on complex medical technology.

Patients in an Intensive Care Department are another special group. An American study states that treatment was withdrawn or withheld in 115 of 1719 admissions to such a department [31]. Of these patients, 89 died in the Intensive Care Department, i.e. 45% of all deaths in this department. Brown studied patients in a nursing home. He reports that 81 of 190 patients with fever did not receive specific treatment and of these 48 died [32].

Withdrawing or withholding treatment upon request of the patient (physician interviews)

During the interviews physicians were asked about situations in which the patient asked explicitly that a life-prolonging treatment be withheld or withdrawn, at least in part with the purpose to shorten life. About half of the physicians indicated they had acceded to such a request at some time. Based on the interviews one can estimate that Dutch physicians annually receive and accede to some 5800 requests of this nature [*]. The reliability of this estimate is less than that of the number of cases of euthanasia. In 80% of the cases of withdrawing and withholding treatment upon request that had occurred most recently and were discussed by the physicians the patient had died in the meanwhile. In almost half the cases the amount of time by which life was shortened was, according to respondents, more than one month. Thus, these decisions can have important consequences in terms of shortening of life. In the opinion of the physicians, the amount of time by which life was shortened due to these decisions is, on the average, greater than was due to euthanasia or assisted suicide.

Withdrawing or withholding treatment without explicit request of the patient (physician interviews)

The decision as to whether a particular treatment can prolong life or contribute to the well-being of a patient, and thus the decision to withdraw or to withhold treatment is part of the daily practice of medicine. Difficult decisions must sometimes be made, e.g. if the chance is small that there will be beneficial consequences, or if life extension can only be achieved at a high cost in terms of pain or invalidity.

In the physician interviews respondents were asked about decisions regarding treatments which could be expected to have a marked life-prolonging effect but which were not carried out without the patient's explicit request to withhold treatment because this effect was not considered desirable or meaningful. These situations are certainly not infrequent. Physicians only gave very general estimates. Based on the interviews one can assume that such decisions are taken in The Netherlands at least 25 000 times annually [*].

In 90% of the latest cases of withdrawing or withholding treatment without explicit request of the patient which were discussed by respondents, the patient had died in the meanwhile. In 16% of the cases hastening the end of life was the

---

[*] This figure should not be compared to the above mentioned number of 22 500 annually because some of these decisions were taken in combination with other MDEL-actions.

Table 17.1   Estimated numbers of MDELs (N.B.: this table can only be interpreted if the text of Chapter 17 is read)[1]

	Physician interviews	Death certificate study	Prospective study	Best estimate
Euthanasia and related MDEL				2.9%
Euthanasia	1.9% (1.6 – 2.2)	1.7% (1.4 – 2.1)	2.6% (2.0 – 3.5)	1.8%
Assisted suicide	0.3% (0.2 – 0.4)	0.2% (0.1 – 0.3)	0.4% (0.2 – 0.9)	0.3%
Life-terminating acts without explicit request	[2]	0.8% (0.6 – 1.1)	1.6% (1.1 – 2.2)	0.8%
The alleviation of pain and/or symptoms, at least taking into account a probable shortening of life	16.3% (15.3 – 17.4)	18.8% (17.9 – 19.9)	13.8% (12.2 – 15.5)	17.5%
Withdrawing or withholding a treatment	[3]	17.9% (17.0- 18.9)	17.0% (15.3 – 18.9)	17.5%
Total MDEL-actions		39.4% (38.1 – 40.7)	35.4% (32.9 – 38.1)	38.0%
DNR-decisions (specialists)	90800 (88500-93200)	59.8% (57.6 – 61.9)	61.4% (56.9 – 66.3)	

1) Percentages refer to total deaths in the Netherlands (128786 in 1990). Numbers refer to all cases for which the particular MDEL was taken, regardless of whether the patient died. The numbers between brackets are the 95% confidence intervals.

2) Material in the physician interviews did not allow computation of this percentage.

3) This percentage in the physician interviews is not comparable with that of the other part-studies because cases of living patients as well as dead patients were discussed.

explicit purpose of the physician. In 58% of cases the patient was totally unable to assess his situation and take a decision adequately and in 21% of cases the patient was not totally able to do so. The extent of life shortening in these cases is much less than when such a decision is taken upon explicit request of the patient. Decisions without explicit request relatively often concern elderly patients (80 years of age and more) for which the distribution of diagnoses does not differ from the distribution of causes of death for The Netherlands. Thus, in such situations, it is not the type of illness that is of great importance, but rather the fact that treatment no longer contributes to the health or well-being of the patient.

Do not resuscitate (DNR) decisions

All physicians were asked during the interview if they ever had taken a DNR decision. All clinical specialists indicated they had taken such a decision at some time. Affirmative answers were given by 40% of nursing home physicians and 21% of general practitioners. These differences are related to different work situations. Almost half the nursing home physicians stated that resuscitation, in principle, is never performed in their nursing home and that therefore a DNR decision is taken implicitly when the patient is admitted. General practitioners frequently work alone. DNR decisions therefore only play a role when the responsibility for the patient (temporarily) is passed on to another physician. We limit ourselves here to the specialists.

In all deaths in which the specialist was the principal treating physician he had taken a DNR decision in about 60% of all deaths (death certificate study 60%, prospective study 61%). This then concerns some 32 000 deaths in the year 1990. Based on the interviews one can estimate that, annually, in hospitals some 91 000 DNR decisions are taken. This implies that such a decision is taken in about 6% of all hospital admissions. In about one third of the cases the patient dies while in hospital. In most cases an MDEL-action also had been performed.

This figure is lower than that reported by Evans for the United States (there are no comparable Dutch figures). Evans reports that a DNR decision is taken for 9% of admissions [33]. Compared to other investigators our figure is somewhat higher: 3% [34] and 2% [35]. In a large scale study of the occurrence of DNR decisions in various Intensive Care Departments Zimmerman found a range from 0.4% to 13.5%. The average was 5.4% [36].

Total percentage of MDEL-actions

Table 17.1 (lowest part) shows that an MDEL-action was performed in 35 to 40% of all deaths (death certificate and prospective studies, 39.4% and 35.4%, respectively). A reasonable estimate is 38%. This amounts to 49 000 deaths in 1990. These figures confirm once more what can be concluded from this entire chapter: MDELs are taken frequently and belong to the normal professional actions of physicians.

18. Summary and conclusions

18.1 Background, design and carrying out of the investigation

Background (Chapter 1)

This report contains the results of an investigation of Medical Decisions concerning the End of Life (MDELs). The investigation was performed upon request of the Commission of Inquiry into the Medical Practice concerning Euthanasia. This commission was installed on 17 January 1990 by the Minister of Justice and the State Secretary of Welfare, Health and Culture.

Although euthanasia has played a central role in the activities of this commission, the investigation was also directed towards other MDELs. The commission formulated the assignment for the investigation as follows:

- The institute (see below for explanation) is requested to investigate and report about the state of affairs with respect to the practice of acting or not acting by a physician with the purpose of hastening the end of life of a patient, whether the patient does, or does not, explicitly requests this. The report will be submitted at a date such that the commission can submit its report to the Minister of Justice and the State Secretary of Welfare, Health and Culture on May 1, 1991.
- The purpose of the investigation is to arrive at a reliable estimate of the number of cases of euthanasia in medical practice (acting to terminate life upon request) and of the number of cases in which life was purposefully terminated, by acts of omissions, without request.
- The investigation should reveal the characteristics of persons for whom euthanasia or termination of life without request was performed, of physicians who are involved and of the decisions that were taken.
- Moreover, the investigation should indicate the extent to which physicians were familiar with the rules of due care when decisions about euthanasia were taken and, if they were familiar with these rules he extent to which, and how, these rules were applied in practice.
- Finally, the conditions have to be studied under which physicians would be prepared to report truthfully that euthanasia or purposeful termination of life without the patient's request was carried out.

The institute mentioned in above assignment was the Department of Public Health and Social Medicine of the Erasmus University in Rotterdam. In addition, the commission has requested the Central Bureau of Statistics to perform a part-study on a sample of death certificates. It was agreed that in addition to this joint report the CBS would also publish independently about their study of death certificates [3].

The project leader for the entire investigation was P.J. van der Maas, M.D., Ph.D., Professor of Public Health and Social Medicine at the Erasmus University, Rotterdam.

Design of the investigation (Chapters 2, 4, 12 and 14)

According to the assignment for the investigation the results of the investigation should not only yield reliable estimates but also provide an insight into the background(s) of decisions. To meet both targets a design was selected that allowed the collection of information about several thousand deaths as well as interviews with several hundred physicians. After extensive consideration it was decided to limit interviews to physicians. Considering the amount of time available this would yield, relatively, a maximum of information.

An investigation design was eventually settled upon which consisted of three parts.

1. A sample of physicians was to be drawn. These physicians were to be approached with the request to participate in an interview (physician interviews).
2. A sample of all deaths over several months was to be drawn. The treating physicians were to be asked to supply in writing information about each deceased concerned; this part of the investigation was to be performed by the CBS (death certificate study).
3. The physicians who were to be interviewed would also be asked to record for a period of half a year a small amount of information for each death in which they had been involved as the treating physician (prospective study).

It was to be expected that certain situations requiring decisions would occur too infrequently to allow any insight to be obtained by this approach. Several experts in appropriate fields were consulted to obtain additional information. These fields, neonatology, other pediatric specialties, psychiatry and AIDS, included patients with special characteristics, e.g. (partly) unable to take a decision, or suffering from diseases with special characteristics (e.g. AIDS).

An extensive questionnaire was used in the physician interviews. In the two other part-studies a brief questionnaire (the "standard questionnaire", length 4 pages, cf. appendix A) was used that could be filled in by the physicians themselves.

A sample of general practitioners, nursing home physicians and specialists was drawn for the interviews. The sample of specialists was derived from specialties most concerned with problems related to the end of life (cardiology, surgery, internal medicine, pulmonology and neurology).

Information was thus obtained that covered 95% of all deaths. The interviews covered patients from the physician's practice for whom an MDEL was made. The interviews, of 406 physicians in total, lasted an average of two and a half hours. The interviews contributed greatly to quantification as well as to gaining an insight into the background(s) of MDELs.

To strengthen the quantitative basis of the investigation a sample was also drawn of individual deaths. The best available base is the causes of death file of the CBS. The size of the sample was set at 8500 cases (Appendix C5). The data in this report are based on 5200 questionnaires returned by physicians. The physicians treating these patients had been asked to fill in the standard questionnaire and to return it to the office of a notary. The data were made completely anonymous and were subsequently analysed by the CBS.

The physicians who had taken part in the interviews were asked to collaborate in the prospective study (see point 3 above). More than 2200 patients were described, using the standard questionnaire.

Concepts and definitions (Chapter 3)

Two concepts are central in this investigation: "Medical Decisions concerning the End of Life (MDELs)" and "MDEL-actions".

In this investigation the term "MDELs" covers all decisions by physicians concerning actions performed with the purpose of hastening the end of life of the patient or actions taking into account the probability that the end of life may be hastened. The actions involved are: withdrawing or withholding treatment (including drip/tube feeding) and the administering, supplying or prescribing of drugs. Also, decisions not to resuscitate (DNR decisions) and the refusal of a request for euthanasia or assisted suicide have been considered in this investigation as an MDEL.

This investigation is not concerned with:

— complications of medical actions or errors, when hastening the end of life of the patient was totally not intended.
— other MDELs, e.g. care of the patient, the possibility to allow the patient to die at home, and all usual medical actions in which (possible) hastening of the end of life is not under consideration.

Considering its defined, limited significance, the term 'Medical Decisions concerning the End of Life' has been capitalised or abbreviated (MDEL) throughout this book.

In the description of the death certificate study and the prospective study (Chapters 13 and 15) the term 'MDEL-action' is used. MDEL-actions are defined as combinations of an action and an intention:

- withdrawing or withholding treatment, either taking into account the probability that this action will hasten the end of life of the patient, or with the explicit purpose of hastening the end of life of the patient;
- intensifying the alleviation of pain and/or symptoms, either taking into account the probability that this action will hasten the end of life of the patient, or, in part with the purpose of hastening the end of life of the patient;
- prescribing, supplying or administering drugs with the explicit purpose of hastening the end of life.

Information about MDEL-actions was collected by means of questions 4 to 7 of the "standard questionnaire" that was used in the death certificate and the prospective studies (Appendix A).

Cooperation in the investigation (Appendix C)

The cooperation of physicians in the studies described in this report was extraordinarily good. Only 9% of the invited physicians refused to participate. Another 2% could not be reached for making an appointment.

In the death certificate study, 76% of the questionnaires sent out were returned. On the whole the questionnaires were filled in carefully and consistently.

Of all physicians interviewed, 80% participated in the prospective study. It appears that these physicians returned questionnaires for virtually all deaths for which they had been the treating physician. The questionnaires were generally completed carefully and consistently in this part of the investigation also.

There were no indications of bias due to selective response in any of the three part-studies.

Results

The most important results are summarised in the sections below. The results of the physician interviews are presented in Chapters 5 to 10, those of the death certificate study in Chapter 13 and those of the prospective study in Chapter 15 and Appendix F. The results of the additional interviews about MDELs for newborns, older children, psychiatric and AIDS patients are described in Chapter 16.

The final estimates of the occurrence of various types of MDELs, as made on the basis of the three part-studies, are presented in Chapter 17.

18.2 Conclusions

The conclusions presented in this chapter are based on a combination of information derived from the three part-studies. Use was also made of the additional interviews and data from the literature. This implies the combining of data from various sources. Choices had thus to be made when assessing what were important or what were less significant results. Although conclusions were considered as carefully as possible it cannot be excluded that the reader of this report will arrive at another interpretation or opinion. Moreover, no attempt was made to be exhaustive when drawing conclusions.

The conclusions drawn are arranged into four groups according to the formulation of the assignment of the investigation.

18.3 The number of cases of euthanasia and other MDELs

Euthanasia and assisted suicide

1. If euthanasia is defined as a the purposeful acting to terminate life by someone other than the person concerned upon request of the latter, euthanasia, to which a physician contributes consciously by prescribing, supplying or administering a drug then occurs in approximately 1.8% of the deaths in The Netherlands. This percentage does not include the withdrawing or withholding of treatment or intensifying the alleviation of pain and/or symptoms with shortening of life as a consequence. For the year 1990 this percentage amounted to 2300 cases of euthanasia, of which 1550 were performed by general practitioners. Euthanasia was performed by a physician in virtually all cases. Euthanasia is sometimes performed by a nurse or someone else, with a drug that was prescribed for this purpose by a physician. In almost all cases the patients whose approaching end of life was hastened were incurably ill. In three quarters of the cases life was shortened by a maximum of four weeks.

2. If assisted suicide is defined as the purposeful assistance of the person concerned to terminate life upon request of the latter, suicide assisted by a physician then occurs annually in about 0.3% of deaths in The Netherlands. This amounted to almost 400 cases for 1990. In almost all cases these were patients in a very advanced stage of an incurable disease. The only difference from euthanasia as described above was that the drug is taken by the patient and not administered by someone else. Shortening of life by more than half a year occurred relatively more often in these cases than with euthanasia. Suicide with the assistance of a physician by persons without an incurable and life-threatening illness is extremely rare.

3. Almost all physicians who treat incurably ill patients are confronted with requests for euthanasia and, less frequently, with requests for assisted suicide. Of all general practitioners 62% at some time performed euthanasia or assisted suicide; this percentage was 44% for specialists, 12% for the nursing home physicians, and 54% for the total for all physicians

participating in this study. Nevertheless, two out of three requests for euthanasia or assisted suicide were not acceded to. Almost all physicians who so far have not performed euthanasia or assisted suicide indicated that they consider it conceivable that they might at some time be prepared to cooperate with an appropriate request. This implies that deciding with regard to, and in part also performing, euthanasia or assisted suicide are important aspects of medical practice.

Other Medical Decisions concerning the End of Life

4. In addition to euthanasia and assisted suicide there are also cases in which life is terminated without explicit request of the patient. Our best estimate is that physicians prescribe, supply or administer a drug with the explicit purpose of hastening the end of life without explicit request of the patient in somewhat more than one thousand cases annually (0.8% of all deaths). In more than half of these cases the decision had been discussed with the patient or the patient had at some time indicated his wish to have the end of life hastened. In several hundreds of cases there was neither discussion with the patient nor a known wish for hastening the end of life.
Virtually all cases involved severely ill or terminal patients who clearly suffered seriously and who were no longer able to make their wishes known. In several cases there had been no consultation with others (family or relatives, colleagues). In a small number of cases there was no consultation while this would have been possible. There were also a small number of cases where life had been shortened by more than half a year and, in the opinion of the physician, the patient clearly had not yet reached the terminal stage of his illness.

5. The investigation showed that some 30% of all deaths in The Netherlands can be described as sudden and unexpected. This implies that in these cases there is, in general, no possibility of taking important medical decisions. One can assume that in almost all other cases there was medical treatment prior to death. Considering the present-day pattern of morbidity in The Netherlands, these cases almost always involved chronic diseases with a shorter or longer course. The investigation showed that in about 38% (35% to 40%) of all deaths one or more MDEL-actions are performed for which the physician at least takes into account the probability that the end of life will be hastened. Such actions may involve withholding or withdrawing treatment(s) or intensifying the alleviation of pain and/or symptoms, particularly using morphine or comparable drugs. There often will be combinations of such actions.
In more than 60% of deaths in which a specialist was the principal treating physician a decision was taken not to resuscitate in case of cardiac or

respiratory arrest. In most of these deaths an MDEL-action was also performed. In addition to these 32 000 do not resuscitate decisions (in 1990, about 53 000 patients died for which a specialist was the treating physician) some 60 000 DNR decisions were taken in hospitals for patients who did not die during the particular admission period. DNR decisions were taken in about 6% of all hospital admissions.

6. The withholding or withdrawing of treatment in cases in which the physician at least takes into account the probability that the end of life will be hastened was the most important MDEL-action in some 17.5% of all deaths. Withholding or withdrawing of treatment can also occur with the explicit purpose of hastening the end of life. This occurred more often than the administration of drugs with the explicit purpose of hastening the end of life. The effect, in terms of life-shortening, is not less, especially not in the case of withholding treatment. In the case of withdrawing or withholding treatment it would perhaps be best to consider this action as refraining from life-prolongation rather than as shortening of life.

7. Intensifying the alleviation of pain and/or symptoms by a physician who uses morphine or similar drugs at doses such that he at least takes into account the probability that the end of life is hastened was a very frequent decision and the most important MDEL-action in 17.5% of deaths. In some of these cases hastening of the end of life was partly the explicit purpose. In the latter case, making a formal distinction between this action and euthanasia or acting to terminate life without explicit request of the patient is not always possible. In addition to situations meeting the definition of euthanasia there are several decisions and actions that can be considered as part of the accepted actions of the medical profession. This boundary area between euthanasia or performing a life-terminating act without specific request on the one hand and intensifying the alleviation of pain and/or symptoms on the other hand can be estimated as including about 2% of all deaths. These 2% are part of the above mentioned 17.5%.

18.4 Characteristics of patients, physicians and situations in which certain decisions were taken

Characteristics of patients

8. There is a clear pattern in the distribution of MDELs according to age, sex and cause of death. The percentage of this kind of decisions for the total number of deaths in a particular age group is about the same for all age groups, being somewhat higher only for the highest age group (80+).
The distribution of the various types of decisions, however, is not similar in the various age groups. Euthanasia and assisted suicide occur mainly in cases

of cancer. Patients are under 65 years of age in about half the cases. The patients are somewhat more often males, contrary to the other MDELs. Men also more often request euthanasia that is not performed.

Intensifying the alleviation of pain and/or symptoms with possible hastening of the end of life occurs relatively less often in the oldest age group (80+). More than half these patients suffer from cancer.

The decision to withhold or withdraw treatment is taken relatively more often with older patients. The distribution of causes of death in these cases does not differ from the distribution found for the total mortality in The Netherlands. It appears that, in such cases, the type of illness is less important than the fact that treatment no longer contributes to the well-being of the patient.

Characteristics of physicians

9. Various types of physicians are faced with MDELs to a varied extent. General practitioners and specialists each took MDELs in over 30% of all deaths for which they had been the treating physicians. The percentages of euthanasia were 2.9% and 1.4% of all deaths for general practitioners and specialists working in hospital, respectively.

   The nursing home physician is confronted relatively more often with MDELs. These MDELs hardly ever relate to euthanasia but mainly to a decision as to withdrawing or withholding treatment.

10. When physicians are classified according to geographical area it appears that in the Western part of The Netherlands ('Randstad') some 60% of physicians stated that they had performed euthanasia at some time. This percentage is about 40% for the other parts of the country.

    Specialists and nursing home physicians were asked about the religious or philosophical orientation of the institution they are affiliated with. The percentage of physicians indicating that they had performed euthanasia at some time was the same for those working in institutions with a religious orientation as for those in other institutions.

Decision-making

11. In cases of euthanasia or assisted suicide the decision had always been discussed with the patient. This finding is tied to the definition of these acts. Life-terminating acts without discussion with or request of the patients almost always concerned patients who are not capable to make a this kind of request.

    The decision to withhold or withdrawn treatment was not discussed with the patient in more than half of the cases. The reason almost always was that, in the opinion of the physician, discussion was not possible.

When the alleviation of pain and/or symptoms was intensified, no discussion with the patient took place in more than half of the cases. In three quarters of the number of patients with whom no discussion had taken place this would not have been possible at the moment that the decision was taken.

12. In 80% of cases of euthanasia and assisted suicide one or more colleagues were consulted. Relatives were consulted in almost all instances.

Concerning the other MDELs, in which there had been discussion with the patient, consultation with a colleague took place in two thirds of all cases. However, a colleague was consulted in about 40% of the cases where the decision had not been discussed with the patient.

18.5 Rules of due care

13. Almost all physicians interviewed were familiar with the existence of rules of due care with respect to euthanasia and they were able to mention one or more of these. Almost all physicians mentioned consultation with one or more colleagues and the carefully considered request was mentioned by two thirds of the physicians. The other rules were mentioned less frequently. However, physicians often said that they would have the rules at their disposal should the need arise.

In cases considered by the physicians themselves as euthanasia or assisted suicide most rules were strictly adhered to (see Section 5.9). The rule that was not met quite often was the keeping of a record of the decision-making process. No written records were available for an average of 40% of the cases. In 16% no colleague was consulted.

Replying to the question as to the importance of the various rules of due care imposed with respect to euthanasia, almost all physicians felt that the voluntariness, the carefully considered request, the unacceptable suffering of the patient, expert information and a technically correct performance were important or very important. Other rules, e.g. the rule for consultation with a colleague was considered important or very important by a smaller percentage of the physicians.

18.6 The reporting procedure

14. The following question was asked during the physician interviews: *"Under what conditions do you feel that one can demand that a physician report a case of euthanasia as a non-natural death to police, coroner or public prosecutor?"*

More than a quarter of physicians felt that euthanasia must always be reported as non-natural death while 22% felt that this could never be asked from a physician.

Physicians were allowed to state more than one condition. A condition put by more than 30% of physicians was that family would not be questioned by police. A quarter of the physicians stated as condition that there would be no prosecution if rules were strictly adhered to.

A condition mentioned by 20% of respondents was a change in procedure, particularly discretion on the part of police. Several of the physicians making such proposals emphasised that they are prepared to report euthanasia but do not wish to be considered as suspects in a criminal act. Also, uncertainty ("I do not know what I will have to go through") is mentioned as an obstacle to reporting non-natural death. Physicians indicated they felt the need for a detailed but clear procedure that would not last for months.

Asked about their opinions concerning several statements made, 94% of respondents felt that, if rules were strictly adhered to, physicians must be able to count absolutely on freedom from prosecution.

18.7 Other conclusions

The investigation

15. The conclusions presented here are based on three part-studies performed in parallel. The results of these studies are consistent on almost all important points. There was excellent collaboration by and openness of the medical profession. There are no indications of important sources of bias. The investigators therefore consider the conclusions presented as valid and reliable.

The future

16. Some expectations for the future can be formulated based on the results of this investigation.

It is certain that, as a consequence of the ageing population the number of deaths per 1000 inhabitants will increase. The average age at death will also increase. It can be expected that with the increase in the number of very old people the number of patients unable to express their own wishes will also increase.

In addition, an important change in the pattern of causes of death is taking place: the proportion of cardiovascular diseases is decreasing and that of cancer is increasing. Considering the distribution of MDELs according to age, sex and cause of death it can be predicted on the basis of demographic and public health developments that the number of MDELs will increase.

A second important aspect is the continuing growth of medical technology. As more possibilities for prolonging life become available the physician will be confronted increasingly often with decisions as to whether to initiate, continue or withhold treatment.

Thirdly there are indications that there is a cultural component in the request for euthanasia and assisted suicide. This investigation showed that requests for euthanasia are fairly frequently made by relatively young people. This also holds for people for whom euthanasia or assisted suicide was performed.

Together, these demographic, public health, medical and cultural developments will cause physicians to be confronted increasingly often with MDELs.

Further development of public opinion

17. Medical decision-making and medical acting concerning the end of life are of good quality in The Netherlands. Nevertheless, there is room for improvement.

This investigation indicates that the development of public opinion within the medical profession and in the various health care sectors can make an important contribution to the quality of medical decisions and actions concerning the end of life. Here are some indications: several respondents indicated after the interview that the interview in itself had made an important contribution to the clarity of their thinking concerning MDELs. Moreover, several respondents indicated during discussion of cases from several years ago that their decision-making would be more thorough in future situations, considering the present-day state of the discussion.

Physicians often stated during the interviews that the present-day openness of the discussion had led to further agreements and procedures for MDELs. In their opinion this often led to a better and more thorough decision-making process. Exceptions were situations in institutions in which a ban was enforced on acts to terminate life. Several physicians reported that this impeded discussion and development of opinions.

19. Epilogue

Introduction

The task of the investigators was limited basically to bringing to light, as well as possible, the facts concerning Medical Decisions concerning the End of Life (MDELs). After one year of intensive contact with the topic and with data obtained and after many discussions with physicians and other experts the investigators developed some ideas that go beyond the results reported in the previous chapters and conclusions. The discussions with the interviewers after the interviews, the extensive case reports made at the end of each interview and the additional interviews brought to light more subtle details than could be presented as straight data in the previous chapters.

Limitations of the investigation

The reasons why physicians exclusively were approached in this investigation were set out in section 2.2. In our opinion, doing this would provide a reliable impression of MDELs in The Netherlands. The limitations, however, are also clear: not all parties concerned with MDELs were consulted. Only indirect information was obtained about the role of nurses. Furthermore, the question as to how relatives experienced the role of the physician and the nurse in an important MDEL cannot be answered. Relatives and nursing staff possibly experienced the decision-making process differently from the physician himself. This topic will be discussed further at the end of this epilogue.

Another important question is whether physicians may have described their role in MDELs too favourably. This possibility can obviously not be excluded. We think, however, that this was the case to, at most, a very limited extent. All interviewers were impressed by the openness shown by most respondents concerning situations in which decisions were taken and about their role in the decision-making process. Almost all respondents felt themselves to have been personally greatly involved in these problems. The possibilities of being able to discuss these matters, with a colleague, under strictest secrecy was very much appreciated by most physicians. In several instances respondents indicated that they would choose a more thorough decision-making process should a given situation occur again.

The manner in which questionnaires in the death certificate and prospective studies were filled in and the additional written information that was often

202

provided also indicated profound involvement and dedication. The various kinds of MDELs will be discussed once more in the following sections.

Withholding or withdrawing treatment

All people are equal in the face of death. This old, reassuring thought has now lost some of its validity. Medieval wood carvings show death taking along the rich and the poor, the young and the old. Even nowadays, death is the most unescapable event in each human life.

There are, however, two important changes that should be reported. The first is that man has succeeded during the past hundred and fifty years in changing his condition in such a way that, in the rich countries, average life expectancy has doubled. The tremendously reduced perinatal and infant mortality made death disappear almost completely from the day-to-day experience of the Dutch and of inhabitants of other rich countries. For inhabitants of poor countries death continues to be a daily reality. It is a fact that life ends with death but the chance of dying at a young age is very unevenly distributed between poor and rich. In this respect not all are equal before death any more.

A second important development is of much more recent date, basically dating only from after World War II: the development of modern medicine. Medicine is obviously increasingly able to assist in curing the sick, in making life bearable for the sick and extending life for a shorter or longer period of time. In other words: death still comes to everyone, but the time when this happens is often partly determined by the decision to withdraw or withhold treatment.

Obviously this does not hold for all deaths. People can die due to accidents or, e.g., an acute myocardial infarction. This investigation showed that about 30% of deaths can be described as sudden and unexpected. In all cases of serious illness, however, physician and patient face the question of whether they should continue therapy or start a new one. It should be considered here that, if people do not die acutely and unexpectedly, death is always preceded by a shorter or longer disease process. The physician is always involved. This is in great contrast with the situation that existed more than a hundred years ago when, e.g., in Amsterdam in more than half of the number of deaths no physician was involved. Medicine must fight death, but not at all costs. Physicians should not act as medical Don Quixotes. Precisely now that medicine can offer so much in terms of prolonging life the task of the physician concerning the end of life is expanding.

In the past, this task primarily involved the provision of adequate terminal care. Increasingly, decision-making by the physician in discussion with the patient and others is among the medical responsibilities concerning the end of life. The decision as to whether to withdraw or withhold treatment increasingly becomes part of terminal care.

Alleviation of pain and symptoms

Medicine has also made progress in the alleviation of symptoms such as severe pain and dyspnea. Morphine and its derivatives can considerably improve the quality of life of patients during long periods of time and in this manner prolong life. The possibilities for a humane and dignified death have greatly increased but there still are limitations. The physician is confronted regularly with the balance between sufficient alleviation of pain and symptoms and shortening of life.

This investigation has shown that intensifying the alleviation of pain and symptoms by using morphine prior to death is not infrequently required and that morphine possibly did shorten the life of the seriously ill or terminal patient in some of such cases. This means that this decision also is an important part of terminal care in many instances.

Euthanasia

The situation just discussed, in which alleviation of pain and symptoms can only be achieved with doses of morphine sufficiently high that they can lead to a shortening of life brings up another aspect of MDELs. There are situations in which life is only suffering, suffering that only ceases when life ceases. The question of medical assistance with hastening the end of life can then be raised. Undoubtedly this question is not a new one. However, it is conceivable that this question will occur more often and possibly more forcefully because of the shift of death towards increasingly higher ages and the increased survival of patients with chronic diseases.

The future

In the future, physicians increasingly will face important MDELs. The reasons were mentioned in Chapter 18:

- mortality increases due to the ageing population;
- the proportion of cancer deaths increases;
- the average age at death increases;
- medical possibilities will develop further.

All this means that, in curative medicine, physicians will be increasingly confronted with questions that concern the end of life and that require a careful decision-making process. This involves the decision not to prolong life or to hasten the end of life; it is not always possible to draw a clear line between these two actions. This decision is made between physician, patient and possibly others who are involved directly. The expertise and integrity of the physician must meet high requirements. It is understandable that society demands guarantees with respect to quality and carefulness for this kind of decision-making, particularly when hastening the end of life is involved. Furthermore, fundamental questions such as if, and on what grounds, a decision may be made to perform a purposeful life-terminating act should always remain the object of public discussion. Patient, physician and society benefit if important aspects of this decision-making process are distinguished and described as clearly as possible. This can contribute to the training of physicians, the communication between the parties concerned and the accountability to society.

One must realise that although a number of characteristics of decisions concerning the end of life can be described clearly and validly, nevertheless, each death is unique and is the completion of the life of one single individual human being. Therefore the quality of MDELs is determined primarily by the human and professional qualities of physician and nurse. The most that can be achieved by setting rules is to provide support in the decision-taking process.

Medical decisions and medical actions concerning the end of life are, on the whole, of good quality in The Netherlands. This quality must be maintained. Improvement is certainly possible. Further open discussion within professional groups and health care sectors can contribute to this improvement. Collegial consultations, also between general practitioner and specialist, can only benefit the quality of decision-making. This holds for patients dying at home as well as those dying in hospital. This kind of consultation will become ever more important. It should be kept in mind that medical possibilities contine to increase and no single physician can be aware of all of them. This will make it increasingly difficult for the individual physician to know whether the possibilities for improving the quality of life for the patient have been exhausted. Furthermore, experience with MDELs plays an important role, which makes it essential for experience to be passed on from teacher to assistant.

Data about the incidence of MDELs are relatively scarce. It is remarkable that attention to various kinds of decisions is rather unevenly distributed. There is a relative abundance of literature about euthanasia in The Netherlands. However, in The Netherlands, decisions to withdraw or withhold treatment and DNR decisions have so far received less attention. This investigation showed that such decisions occur relatively frequently and can have important consequences. The attention of physicians and investigators could be spread more evenly over various types of MDELs.

MDELs should have a distinct place in the medical education and in further professional training. This is also true for the training of other professionals in health care. Every physician should have available sufficient knowledge and possibilities for consulting others and for achieving a careful decision-making process, regardless of the outcome of thisprocess. Communication between physician and patient and possibly others demands particular attention. Research has shown that physicians often underestimate the communication gap between physician and patient. Great effort and investment of time are required from the physician to achieve a joint decision between patient and physician in situations in which important medical decisions are taken. This certainly holds for MDELs, which often are complicated and emotion-laden. Patience and carefulness in discussions with the patient is an obvious requirement. Consultation with relatives must be of the same quality. Relatives must have no feeling of grief or reproach that could have been avoided by better communication.

Physicians must be prepared to account for their decisions and actions with respect to profound decisions concerning the end of life. This investigation showed that they are indeed prepared to do so. There should be no secrecy around MDELs, but the intimacy between the patient, other persons involved and the physician must be maintained under all circumstances.

Rotterdam, August 1991.

References

1 State committee on euthanasia, Report on euthanasia (in Dutch), Government Printing Office, The Hague, 1985.

2 Blad, J.R., Between blind fate and self-determination (in Dutch), Gouda Quint, Arnhem, 1990.

3 Central Bureau of Statistics, The end of life in medical practice; findings of a survey sampled from deaths occuring July–November 1990, SDU, The Hague, 1992.

4 Maas, P.J. van der, Medical decisions concerning the end of life, investigation commissioned by the Remmelink committee (in Dutch), Nederlands Tijdschrift voor Geneeskunde, 134 (1990) 1802–1805.

5 Royal Dutch Medical Association, Position statement on euthanasia (in Dutch), Royal Dutch Medical Association, Utrecht, 1984.

6 Leenen, H.J.J., Handbook on health law (in Dutch), Samson, Alphen a/d Rijn, 1988.

7 Delden, J.J.M. van, Foregoing medical treatments in incompetent adults (in Dutch), Health Council, The Hague, 1991.

8 Royal Dutch Medical Association, Discussion paper on life-terminating acts in incompetent patients, Part II: Permanent comateus patients (in Dutch), Royal Dutch Medical Association, Utrecht, 1991.

9 Wijmen, F.C.B. van, Physicians and the self-chosen ending of life (in Dutch), State University of Limburg, Maastricht, 1989.

10 Health Council, Recommendations concerning euthanasia in neonates (in Dutch), Government Printing Office, The Hague, 1975.

11 Dutch Pediatric Society, Act or not act (in Dutch), NVK, 1988.

12 Royal Dutch Medical Association, Interim report on life-terminating acts in incompetent patients, Part I: Severely handicapped neonates (in Dutch), Royal Dutch Medical Association, Utrecht, 1990.

13 Health Council, Suicide (in Dutch), Health Council, The Hague, 1986.

14 Dutch Right to Die Society, Committee of assisstance for questions concerning suicide, Report on assistance in questions concerning suicide (in Dutch), NVVE, Amsterdam, 1991.

15 Boom, F. van den, Grimmen, T., Mead, C., Rozenburg, H., AIDS, euthanasia and distress, Sixth International Conference on AIDS, Florence, 1991.

16 Wal, G. van der, Eijk, J.Th.M. van, Leenen, H.J.J., Spreeuwenberg, C., Euthanasia and assisted suicide performed by physicians in general practice (in Dutch), Medisch Contact, 46 (1991) 174–176.

17 Wal, G. van der, Christ, L.M., Schuyt-Lucassen, N.Y., Ribbe, M.W., Eyk, J.Th.M. van, Euthanasia and assisted suicide performed by nursing home physicians (in Dutch), Medisch Contact, 46 (1991) 1039–1041.

18 Kuhse, H., Voluntary euthanasia in the Netherlands, Medical Journal of Australia, 147 (1987) 394–396.

19 Angell, M., Euthanasia, New England Journal of Medicine, 319 (1988) 1348–1350.

20 British Medical Association, Euthanasia, BMA, London, 1988.

21 Vos, M., Reporting of euthanasia (in Dutch), Medisch Contact, 40 (1985) 1059–1060.

22 Fenigsen, R., Mercy, murder and morality perspectives on euthanasia, A case against Dutch euthanasia, Hastings Center Report, 19 (1989) 22–30.

23 Schudel, W.J., Euthanasia (request) (in Dutch), Epidemiologisch bulletin GG&GD, GG&GD, The Hague, 1987.

24 Bartelds, A.I.M., Fracheboud, J., Zee, J. van der, The Dutch sentinal practice network; relevance for public health policy, NIVEL, Utrecht, 1989.

25 Wal, G. van der, Eijk, J.Th.M. van, Leenen, H.J.J., Spreeuwenberg, C., Euthanasia and assisted suicide performed by physicians with patients treated at home, I Diagnosis, age and sex of patients (in Dutch), Nederlands Tijdschrift voor Geneeskunde, 135 (1991) 1593–1598.

26 Wal, G. van der, Eijk, J.Th.M. van, Leenen, H.J.J., Spreeuwenberg, C., Euthanasia and assisted suicide performed by physicians with patients treated at home, II Suffering by the patient (in Dutch), Nederlands Tijdschrift voor Geneeskunde, 135 (1991) 1599–1603.

27 Oliemans, A.P., Nijhuis, H.G.J., Euthanasia in general practice (in Dutch), Medisch Contact, 41 (1986) 691.

28 GG&GD, The Amsterdam sentinal practice network project (in Dutch), Annual report 1986, GG&GD, Amsterdam, 1987.

29 Neu, S., Kjellstrand, C.M., Stopping long-term dialysis. An empirical study of withdrawal of life-supporting treatment, New England Journal of Medicine, 314 (1986) 14–20.

30 Nieuwkerk, C.M.J. van, Krediet, R.T., Arisz, L., Voluntary termination of dialysis by chronic dialysis patients (in Dutch), Nederlands Tijdschrift voor Geneeskunde, 134 (1990) 1549–1552.

31 Smedira, N.G., Evans, B.H., Grais, L.S., et al., Withholding and withdrawal of life support from the critically ill, New England Journal of Medicine, 322 (1990) 309–315.

32 Brown, N.K., Thompson, D.J., Nontreatment of fever in extended-care facilities, New England Journal of Medicine, 300 (1979) 1246–1250.

33 Evans, A.L., Brody, B., The DNR order in teaching hospitals, Journal of the American Association, 253 (1985) 2236–2239.

34 Lipton, H., DNR decisions in a community hospital, Journal of the American Association, 256 (1986) 1164–1169.

35 Bedell, S.E., Pelle, D., Maher, P.L., Cleary, P.D., DNR orders for critically ill patients in the hospital. How are they used and what is their impact?, Journal of the American Association, 256 (1986) 233–237.

36 Zimmerman, J.E., Knaus, W.A., Sharpe, S.M., Anderson, A.S., Draper, E.A., Wagner, D.P., The use and implications of DNR orders in ICU's, Journal of the American Association, 255 (1986) 351–356.

Additional references

This additional bibliography lists those sources that we have found to be especially useful or thought-provoking. We do not attempt to list all of the many articles, books, and other documents currently available on these topics.

American Medical Association, Council on Ethical and Judicial Affairs, Decisions near the end of life, Journal of the American Medical Association, 67 (1992) 2229–2233.

Blackhall, L.J., Must we always use CPR? New England Journal of Medicine, 317 (1987) 1281–1285.

Emanuel, E.J., A review of the ethical and legal aspects of terminating medical care, American Journal of Medicine, 84 (1988) 291–301.

Hastings Center The, Guidelines on the termination of life-sustaining treatment and the care of the dying. The Hastings Center, Briarcliff Manor, NY, 1987.

McCormick, R.A., To save or to let die: the dilemma of modern medicine, Journal of the American Medical Association, 229 (1974) 172–176.

Office of Technology Assessment, Life-sustaining technologies and the elderly, OTA-BA-306, Government printing office, Washington DC, 1987.

President's commission for the study of ethical problems in medicine and biomedical and behavioral research, Deciding to forego life-sustaining treatment, Government Printing Office, Washington DC, 1983.

Singer, P.A. and Siegler, M., Elective use of life-sustaining treatments in internal medicine, Advances in Internal Medicine, 36 (1991) 57–79.

Tomlinson, T. and Brody, H., Ethics and communication in Do-Not-Resuscitate orders, New England Journal of Medicine, 318 (1988) 43–46.

Wanzer, S.H., Federman, D.D., Adelstein, S.J. et al., The physician's responsibility toward hopelessly ill patients, A second look, New England Journal of Medicine, 320 (1989) 844–849.

Weir, R.F., Abating treatment with critically ill patients, Oxford University Press, New York, 1989 (esp. Chapter 6: 'Options among ethicists').

Appendices

The Standard Questionnaire   Appendix A

1.	In respect of this death, where you acting as:	0 specialist/specialist-in-training/ assistant-physician- not-in-training 0 general practitioner/general practitioner-in-training 0 nursing home physician/trainee nursing home physician 0 in a different function to those named above
2.	When was your first contact with the patient?	0 before or at the time of death –> go to question **3** 0 after death –> go to question **24**
3.	Was death sudden and totally unexpected?	0 yes –> go to question **22** 0 no –> go to question **4**
4.	Did you or a colleague take one or more of the following actions, or ensure that one of them was taken, <u>taking into account the probability</u> that this action would hasten the end of the patient's life: (please reply to all three questions, 4a, 4b and 4c)	
4a	withholding a treatment*?	0 yes 0 no
4b	withdrawing a treatment *?	0 yes 0 no
4c	intensifying the alleviation of pain and/or symptoms using morphine or a comparable drug?	0 yes –> go to question **5** 0 no –> go to question **6**
5.	Was hastening the end of life <u>partly the purpose</u> of the action indicated in question 4c?	0 yes 0 no
6.	Was death caused by one or more of the following actions, which you or a colleague decided to take <u>with the explicit purpose</u> of hastening the end of life: (answer both 6a and 6b)	
6a	withholding a treatment*?	0 yes 0 no
6b	withdrawing a treatment*?	0 yes 0 no

*   In this study, 'treatment' is taken to include 'tube feeding'

7. Was the death caused by the use of a drug** prescribed, supplied or administered by you or a colleague <u>with the explicit purpose</u> of hastening the end of life (or of enabling the patient to end his own life)?

0 yes
0 no

If yes, who administered this drug** (= introduced it into the body)? (tick one or more answers)

0 the patient himself in the doctor's presence
0 the patient himself without the doctor being present
0 you or a colleague
0 a nurse
0 another person in the doctor's presence
0 another person without the doctor being present

If <u>at least one</u> of the items of questions 4, 5, 6 and 7 was answered with **"yes"**, go to question **8**.

If <u>all</u> parts of questions 4, 5, 6 and 7 were answered with **"no"**, go to question **22**.

Questions 8 to 21 relate to the <u>last "yes" in answer to questions 4 to 7</u>.

8. A question about that (last mentioned) action: In your estimation, by how much was the life of the patient in fact shortened by this action?

0 more than six months
0 one to six months
0 one to four weeks
0 up to one week
0 less than 24 hours
0 life probably was not shortened at all

9. Did you or a colleague discuss with the patient the (possible) hastening of the end of life as a result of the last-mentioned action?

0 yes, at the time of performing the action or shortly before—> go to question 10
0 yes, some time beforehand (and not at the time of, or shortly before) –> go to question 10
0 yes, I do not know when – > go to question 10
0 no, no discussion –> go to question 16

10. Who took the initiative to discuss the situation with the patient? (tick one ore more answers)

0 the patient
0 you or a colleague
0 nursing staff
0 the patient's partner
0 (other) relatives of the patient
0 pastor, spiritual adviser
0 other persons
0 do not know

11. At the time of the <u>discussion,</u> did you consider the patient able to assess his/her situation and to take a decision about it adequately?

0 yes
0 no, not or not totally able

12. Was the decision concerning the (last-mentioned) action taken upon an explicit request of the patient?

0 yes –> go to question 13
0 no –> go to question 15

** This may mean one or more drugs; morphine is also sometimes used for this purpose.

13. At the time of this <u>request</u>, did you consider the patient able to assess his/her situation and take a decision about it adequately?

0 yes
0 no, not or not totally able

14. Did the patient express this request repeatedly?

0 yes

15a. Was there a written advance directive available?

0 yes –> go to question **15b**
0 no –> go to question **21**

15b Did this play part in reaching the decision?

0 yes –> go to question **21**
0 no –> go to question **21**

Only answer questions 16 to 20 if the answer to question 9 was "no, no discussion"

16. Was it possible to discuss the situation with the patient at the time when the (last-mentioned) action was decided upon?

0 yes
0 no

17. Why was this decision not discussed with the patient?
(tick one or more answers)

0 patient was too young
0 patient was too emotionally unstable
0 this (last-mentioned) action was clearly the best one for the patient
0 discussion would have done more harm than good
0 patient was temporarily unconscious
0 patient was permanently unconscious
0 patient was in a state of diminished consciousness
0 patient was demented
0 patient was mentally handicapped
0 patient was suffering from a psychiatric disorder
0 other, if you wish you may expand on this at question **24**

18. Did one of the following make an explicit request to hasten the patient's life:
(tick one or more answers)

0 partner of patient
0 parents of patient
0 guardian, or authorized representative of patient
0 children of patient
0 (other) relatives of the patient
0 colleague
0 nursing staff
0 others
0 no explicit request

19. As far as you know, did the patient ever express a wish for the end of life to be hastened?

0 yes –> go to question **20**
0 no –> go to question **21**

20. How were you informed of this wish?
(tick one or more answers)

0 verbally by the patient
0 by a written directive of the patient
0 verbally by a colleague
0 in writing by a colleague
0 by relatives or other persons
0 otherwise, if you wish you may expand on this at question **24**

21. Did you or a colleague discuss with
    anybody else the (possible) hastening
    of the end of the patient's life before
    it was decided to take the last-mentioned
    action that was indicated by **"yes"**
    in questions **4 to 7?**
    (tick one or more answers)

0 with one or more colleagues
0 nursing staff
0 partner of patient
0 (other) relatives of patient
0 pastor, spiritual adviser
0 guardian, authorized representative of patient
0 other persons
0 nobody

22. Did you or a colleague clearly
    agree in advance that in the event
    of a (functional) cardiac and/or
    respiratory arrest no attempt would
    be made to resuscitate this patient?
    (a so-called Do Not Resuscitate decision)?
    (tick one or more answers)

0 yes, with other doctors
0 yes, with nursing staff
0 yes, with the patient
0 yes, with relatives of the patient
0 not explicitly for this patient; however, implicitly
   based on the agreement that resuscitation will not
   in general be attempted in our institution
0 no

23. Was there an explicit request
    to terminate life that
    was not carried out?
    (tick one or more answers)

0 no, there was no explicit request that was not
   carried out
0 yes, request by patient
0 yes, request by relatives
0 yes, request by other persons

24. If in your opinion your answers to the questions would benefit from further clarification, please provide this in the space below

Documents used for the investigation

Appendix B

B.1 Letter from the chief inspector of the health supervisory service and the chairman of the royal dutch medical association to all physicians (± 30 000) in the Netherlands

Rijswijk, 13 August 1990

Subject: Investigation "Medical actions concerning the end of life"; request for cooperation

Dear Colleague,

In the coming months a great number of physicians will be approached with the request to collaborate in an investigation of medical decisions concerning the end of life. The investigation is to be performed by the Department of Public Health and Social Medicine of the Erasmus University in Rotterdam and the Central Bureau of Statistics in Voorburg. The purpose of this joint letter is to describe briefly the background of this investigation.

On 18 January 1990 the Minister installed the Commission of Inquiry into the Medical Practice concerning euthanasia, referred to in the media as the "Remmelink Commission". The task of this Commission is to report to the Minister of Justice and the State Secretary of Welfare, Health and Culture. For this purpose the Remmelink Commission is sponsoring a study of the state of affairs concerning the practice of acting, or not acting, by a physician with the purpose of hastening the end of life of a patient, on his explicit request, or not. The investigation is therefore broader than the term 'euthanasia' would suggest.
The investigation consists of several parts.

A carefully drawn sample of physicians will be asked to collaborate with a structured interview in which the factual course of actions as well as the considerations that led to a particular decision will be discussed. These physicians will also be asked to record, during a period of six months and for the purpose of this study, some data concerning all deaths occurring during the period in which they are involved as treating physician.

This part of the study is to be carried out by the Department of Public Health and Social Medicine at the Erasmus University in Rotterdam, under direction of Prof. Dr. P.J. van der Maas.

Furthermore a sample of deaths will be drawn from the files managed by the medical officer of the Central Bureau of Statistics. The physician who acted as treating physician for a particular patient will be asked to provide further information concerning the end of life of the patient.
This part of the study is to be carried out by the Central Bureau of Statistics (CBS).

Utmost care will be taken to protect the privacy of the physicians and the relatives of the deceased. The CBS will collect its information in writing and completely anonymously. The information supplied to the CBS will not be usable to trace back either physician or deceased. The interview data obtained by Erasmus University will be made anonymous immediately upon its receipt. The possibility of indirect identification is also excluded.
The information supplied will not be used for any other purpose than to answer the questions raised by this investigation. The investigation will have no legal consequences for any of the participants.

The physicians selected for this study will be informed in detail about the manner in which the data will be handled.
Considering the large size of both samples it is not impossible that some physicians will be involved with the investigation more than once, e.g. because they are invited to participate in an interview, while at the same time the CBS may ask them one or more times to provide information about one or more deaths. There is no question of "double work", because this concerns two independent parts of the investigation. The results will only be brought together when the report is produced. The data required are purposely collected and analysed separately and therefore can never be traced to one particular respondent.

Considering the great social importance of this investigation we jointly appeal to you for your collaboration should one of the two institutes mentioned approach you to ask that you participate in the investigation.

(was signed by)
The Chief Inspector of the Health Supervisory Service
The Chairman of the Royal Dutch Medical Association

B.2 Letter from prof. P.J. van der Maas, M.D., Ph.D., project leader, to physicians of the interview study

Rotterdam, October 1990

Dear Colleague........,

You probably know that an investigation has now been started about medical decisions concerning the end of life upon request of the "Commission of Inquiry into the Medical Practice concerning Euthanasia", chaired by Prof. Dr. J. Remmelink.

The purpose of the study is to arrive at a reliable estimate of the number of cases of euthanasia (life-terminating acts upon request) and of purposely performing a life-terminating act not upon request, in medical practice. The aim of this investigation therefore goes further than euthanasia: other decisions concerning the end of life will also be studied.

Within the framework of this investigation 400 physicians will be interviewed about ther experiences with and their opinions about medical decisions concerning the end of life. Among these 400 physicians there will be general practitioners, nursing home physicians and specialist clinicians. We obtained your address in the course of the drawing of a random sample.

Thus you are one of the 400 physicians we should like to interview for this study. You will therefore be telephoned in the near future by our colleague, ..., M.D. to make an appointment.
The nature of the investigation requires that interviews with specialists should be held with persons who have been active clinically for a minimum of two years in the same institution. We do not know whether you belong to this category. If you do not, would you please let us know as soon as possible? Our telephone number is given at the end of this letter.

I should like to point out, perhaps unnecessarily, that the scientific and social usefulness of the results of this investigation depends on a good response from the medical profession. Even if, in your opinion, you have never taken a serious decision concerning the end of life of a patient or if you have serious objections to euthanasia it is of great importance for us to be permitted to hear about your experiences and opinions. I should like to refer you to the enclosed letter of recommendation from the Chief Inspector of the Health Supervisory Service and the Chairman of the Royal Dutch Medical Association. In due course you will receive a copy of the complete report as sign of gratitude for your cooperation.

Maximal care will be given to your privacy and that of the relatives. The data will be made anonymous immediately upon receipt. Moreover, no one will be able to claim the data and the data will not be used for any purpose other than to answer the questions raised by this investigation. The interviewer will hand you a description of the procedure used to safeguard secrecy.

Should you be interested, my collaborators and I would be pleased to provide further information. We can be reached by telephone, on 010-4087714.

I trust that you will be prepared to cooperate with this study.
Yours very truly,

(was signed)
Prof. P.J. van der Maas, M.D., Ph.D.
Projectleader

B.3 Letter from L.M. Friden-Kill, M.D., medical officer, Central Bureau of Statistics, to physicians of the death certificate study

Dear Colleague,

The CBS has been invited to collaborate in the investigation *'Medical Decisions concerning the End of Life'*, organised on request of the *Commission of Inquiry into the Medical Practice concerning Euthanasia*, the Remmelink Commission. The purpose of the investigation is summarised in the enclosed letter by the Chief Inspector of the Health Supervisory Service and the Chairman of the Royal Dutch Medical Association. The study performed by the CBS is based on a sample of death certificates (B forms). The study concerns persons who died in the period July to November 1990.

In connection with this study I should like to ask you to reply to several questions by marking the appropriate answering categories which relate to a death that is part of the sample. As far as I could ascertain it concerns one of your patients. Your and your patient's anonymity are guaranteed by a special procedure that also involves a notary.

To indicate the death involved I can supply the following data:

Municipality where death occurred..............
Number of death certificate................
Date of birth..........................
Date of death..........................
Sex ....
Municipality where the deceased resided.....
Sample number...........................

The name and address of the deceased are not known to me. Based on the number of the death certificate, the officer responsible for the population registry in the municipality where death occurred can inform you of the deceased's name.

For the purpose of the study I am sending you:

1. an anonymous questionnaire.
2. a *large brown* envelope marked with the sample number stated above.
3. a *large white* envelope addressed to Mr. Mulder, notary at The Hague.
4. a *small brown* envelope addressed to the CBS.

Please be kind enough to fill in the questionnaire (1) and put it into the large brown envelope (2). After sealing please put the sealed brown envelope (containing the filled-in questionnaire) into the white envelope and mail the sealed white envelope to the notary. The notary will remove the sample number from the brown envelope and thereafter hand the unopened envelope to me.

If you *were not the treating physician* and therefore cannot reply to the questions nor can have them answered conveniently, please return this letter directly to me in the small brown envelope (4) provided, mentioning the name of the treating physician. The remaining material can be destroyed.

The procedure described above is part of the procedures to safeguard the data of this investigation. It will not be possible to discover the name of the respondent to a questionnaire or the name of the deceased, either on the way to, or within, the CBS. This guarantees complete anonymity. Upon request, I can provide further written information about the safeguarding procedures, including a copy of the protocol signed by the notary.

Further information about the procedures followed and other questions, e.g. the filling in of the questionnaire can be obtained from the research team of the CBS: 070-3694341, ext. 2905.

Considering the rather large size of the sample it is possible that I shall ask you again in the near future to fill in our questionnaire regarding deaths in which you were concerned as the treating physician. I should be most grateful if you would then again be prepared to cooperate.

I thank you for your cooperation.

Yours very truly,
L.M. Friden - Kill, M.D.
Medical Officer

Sampling, response and representativity

Appendix C

C.1 Introduction

It was important for the success of the investigation that the response to each of the part-studies would be sufficiently high and that the results could be considered as representative for the physicians in The Netherlands. In this appendix there is first some background information of the sampling procedures for the physician interviews and the prospective study. The response to, and the representativity of the three part-studies will be discussed thereafter.

C.2 The sample of physicians

Table C.1 presents a summary of the distribution of the deaths that occurred in hospital, subdivided according to the specialties included in the sample of physicians. The table shows that physicians from the five specialties selected (cardiology, surgery, internal medicine, pulmonology and neurology) are involved as the most important treating physician in 89% of hospital deaths. It should be mentioned that this registry is not entirely complete because patients dying before their "administrative admission to hospital" (e.g. due to accidents or myocardial infarction) are not included. We assumed that these acute deaths were distributed proportionally among the specialties.

Table C.1   Hospital deaths in 1989, subdivided according to specialties[1])

Specialty	Deceased n=48525 %
Cardiology	15.5
Surgery	12.6
Internal medicine	38.5
Pulmonology	9.8
Neurology	12.4
Other specialties	11.2
Total	100.0

1)   Source: Dutch Centre for Health Care Information (SIG)

The further distribution of deaths in The Netherlands will be discussed in Appendix E. It can be stated here that general practitioners, nursing home physicians and the five specialties selected are, together, involved in 95% of all deaths in The Netherlands.

C.3 Response to physician interviews

Much effort was put into maximizing the response. In Section 2.10 the steps taken to obtain maximal cooperation from the medical profession were discussed.

When arrangements were made, the majority of respondents selected were immediately prepared to agree to an interview, this in spite of the advance communication that they would have to reserve at least 1½ hours. Other physicians agreed only after some hesitation.

Table C.2 summarises the response obtained for the physician interviews. A total of 599 addresses was selected. It appeared later that 138 of these did not meet the selection criteria; the reasons are listed in Table C.5. The reasons for "participation impossible" are also shown in Table C.5. Of 447 physicians meeting the selection criteria and qualifying for participation 41 refused, resulting in an average refusal percentage of 9%.

Of the three groups of respondents the nursing home physicians were the most cooperative, followed by the general practitioners (Table C.2). The percentage of refusals by specialists was subdivided into specialties. It is noteworthy that cardiologists and internists refused more than average and surgeons, pulmonologists and neurologists less than average (Table C.3).

Table C.2   Response to physician interviews

	General practitioner	Specialist	Nursing home physician	Total
Intended number of interviews	150	210	50	410
a. total of addresses selected	173	352	74	599
b. did not meet criteria	6	109	23	138
c. met criteria (a – b)	167	243	51	461
d. participation impossible	3	11	0	14
e. participation possible (c – d)	164	232	51	447
f. refusals	12	28	1	41
g. % refusals (f/e x 100)	7%	12%	2%	9%
h. interviews performed	152	204	50	406
i. of which unusable	0	1	0	1

The reasons for refusal are listed in Table C.4. The most frequently heard reason was "no time". We asked the respondent to free 1½ hours in any case for the interview. In a small number of cases it was agreed with the respondent that the interview would be limited to one hour. The time spent often became longer. The average duration of an interview was 2½ hours. The second most frequently mentioned reason for refusal was the great political charge of the topic or insufficient confidence in the anonymity guarantees.

The refusing physicians were asked to reply to several questions in a telephone interview; this was agreed to in 17 of 41 cases (41%). The analysis of replies on this so-called no-response list does not suggest that the refusals came from a certain type of respondent. Thus there are no indications that the no-response group belongs to a particular selection.

Several respondents appeared not to belong to the intended group of respondents after telephone contact had been made (Table C.5). Some had retired, some had not yet spent two years working in their practice or were not (no longer) active in the clinic. Some specialists no longer belonged to their initial specialty (e.g. a neurologist who had become a physician in a mother and child health centre) or were active in psychiatry or paediatrics, specialties which were approached in a different manner.

C.4 Representativity of physician interviews

Section 4.2 described the procedure followed in cases when an intended respondent refused or later appeared not to meet selection criteria. In brief, in case of refusal another respondent was selected within the same age group and

Table C.3   Refusals subdivided according to specialties (physician interviews)

Specialisme	Total number	Absolut number refusals specialists	Refusals %
Cardiologists	34	9	21%
Surgeons	34	3	8%
Internists	68	13	16%
Pulmonologists	34	1	3%
Neurologists	34	2	6%
Total	204	28	12%

Table C.4   Reasons for refusal (physician interviews)

	General practitioner	Specialist	Nursing home physician
No time (too busy, interview takes too long, etc.)	5	13	1
Opposed to study (only political, not anonymous, etc.)	1	9	–
Never participate in enquiries	–	2	–
No comment	–	4	–
Already participated in North Holland (van der Wal) study	1	–	–
No time – against euthanasia/euthanasia does not occur in his/her practice	2	–	–
Recent illness/partly unable to work	3	–	–
Total	12	28	1

province of practice, while in the case of selection criteria not being met another 'aselect' respondent was selected within the same province. No source of bias is introduced, in principle, by this procedure. Table C.2 shows that the selected general practitioners almost all met the selection criteria because an up to date file was used of the Dutch Institute for Primary Health Care (NIVEL). Most of the replacements of nursing home physicians in the sample were due to the fact that many respondents had not yet been working in the same institution for two years.

The most important problem occurred with respect to the file of specialists (file of the Supervisory Health Service (GHI)). This file was not always up to date with respect to closing of the practice, change of professional activity or specialty, etc. This is apparent from Table C.5.

The same replacement procedure was followed for a total of 20 physicians with whom no appointment could be made as for those who did not meet selection criteria (see Table C.5). Also here it is not likely that any bias arose in the composition of the group of respondents.

An important question is whether the refusers form a select group such that this could lead to important bias. Considering the total number of refusals this can hardly be the case. Moreover, the reasons for refusal are various (see Table C.4). Only the total of 15 refusers who indicated that they were not in favour of this investigation, who did not wish to comment or stated that they opposed euthanasia could introduce a very modest bias.

Taking into account all relevant information we see no reason to assume that refusals introduced any bias.

Table C.5   Did not meet selection criteria/participation impossible (physician interviews)

	General practitioner	Specialist	Nursing home physician	Total
Did not meet selection criteria				
Working abroad	–	5	–	5
Retired	4	22	4	30
Not working in hospital	–	41	6	47
Not yet two years in same practice/institution	1	16	13	30
"Wrong" specialty	–	24	–	24
Deceased	1	1	–	2
Total	5	109	23	138
Participation not possible				
Long-standing illness	3	7	–	10
Cannot be found	–	4	–	4
Total	3	11	–	14

C.5 Response in the death certificate study

The following background data were available from the sample of the deceased: stratum number, age, sex, cause of death and place of death. Based on the sample, estimates can be made of the population of deceased persons subdivided according to combinations of the above-mentioned criteria, taking into account the sampling design. The differences found in the sampling fractions were balanced by assigning weights to the elements in the sample which were the reciprocals of the sampling fractions. The weights for the strata from 1 to 4 then have the values 12, 8, 4 and 2.

Stratum 0 was not observed. This stratum is of no importance for the analysis of and the correction for non-response. A small number of questionnaires received for the other strata could not be used or were filled in insufficiently. This "unusable response" was eventually counted as non-response. In this sub-section the response percentages were calculated by weighting the usable response with the reciprocal of the sampling fraction and expressing this value as percent of the weighted sample. Stratum 0 was not considered here. Table C.6 gives an impression of the structure of the population and of the response, excluding stratum 0.

The differences between the response percentages for men and women are minimal. However, the differences between response percentages related to those deceased in hospital and elsewhere are considerable. One of the explanations for the higher non-response for hospitals is the difficulty physicians in hospitals have in certain cases in discovering what patient was involved. The differences between response percentages for different age groups were generally low. Relatively speaking, there were somewhat larger differences for small population sizes. However, for such cases the sample size was also small (the sampling fraction was about 1 in 6). So in some

Table C.6   Estimated population size with its response percentages according to age, sex, cause of death, stratum (excluding stratum 0) and place of death, based on the sample drawn. Period: August to November 1990 (death certificate study)

	Place of death				Place of death		
	Hospital	Elsewhere	Total		Hospital	Elsewhere	Total
	Absolute numbers				Response percentage		
Total	16,742	20,258	36,730		64	81	73
Age							
0 year	192	60	252		77	53	71
01-11	28	36	64		86	89	88
12-19	56	24	80		79	83	80
20-49	878	678	1,556		69	74	71
50-64	2,652	2,308	4,960		63	82	72
65-79	7,282	6,806	14,088		64	82	73
80+	5,384	10,346	15,730		65	80	75
Sex							
Male	8,734	9,634	18,368		64	82	74
Female	7,738	10,624	18,362		65	79	73
Primary cause of death							
Cancer	4,896	6,944	11,840		65	81	74
Cardiovascular diseases	5,178	5,338	10,516		63	81	72
Nervous system	1,948	2,688	4,636		67	83	76
Pulmonary diseases	1,204	1,746	2,950		64	78	72
External causes	262	136	398		62	74	66
Mental disorders	52	262	314		92	79	82
Others	2,336	2,298	4,634				
Stratum							
1	3,828	3,360	7,188		64	79	71
2	5,216	6,152	11,368		63	79	72
3 and 4	7,428	10,746	18,040		66	82	75

subgroups one respondent more or less can make a difference of more than 10%.

Also there are only small differences between different causes of death, particularly for the most important causes of death. Also the differences in response percentages per stratum are small.

Table C.6 shows that the place of death is the most important response percentage variable that can contribute to an explanation of differences. The response percentage was very high for those deaths not occurring in hospital. There were no important differences for men and women and for various age groups as long as the response percentages were based on sufficiently large numbers of respondents. Important differences also could not have been expected because it is not likely that the physician's response depended on the age and sex of the deceased. It is important that the response percentage depended very little on cause of death and stratum because these characteristics are strongly related to the incidence of MDEL-actions.

The weighted response percentage of 73% for the total is somewhat less than the 76% for the unweighted percentage of questionnaires returned. The difference is due in part to the weighting procedure. Furthermore, the unusable questionnaires were not counted into the final response.

C.6 Response, completeness and representativity in the prospective study

Table C.7 presents a summary of the response by different groups of physicians in the prospective study. Response here means the percentage of physicians interviewed that participated in the prospective study regardless of whether one or more deaths occurred in the period of participation. This percentage could be established accurately.

The table shows the initial number of participants, the number of participants who eventually supplied information and the total of "physician-weeks" upon which the results of the prospective study were based. A "physician-week" is a week during which one particular respondent cooperated with the prospective study regardless of whether, or not, a death occurred. Although most physicians indicated after the interview that they would be prepared to participate in the prospective study, actual participation was unevenly distributed over the different specialties. In particular, several specialists working in hospitals stated sooner or later that they saw no way of

Table C.7 **Response for the prospective study[1]**

	Number of respondents interviewed	Number of prospective participants	Eventual participants in prospective study	Total "physician- weeks"	Expected number of deaths	Number of deaths described
General practitioners	152	146	138 (91%)	3399	568	618 (109%)
Cardiologists	34	28	22 (65%)	459	210	267 (127%)
Surgeons	34	31	24 (71%)	541	97	102 (105%)
Internists	68	56	43 (63%)	892	362	378 (104%)
Pulmonologists	33	29	26 (79%)	602	241	257 (107%)
Neurologists	34	31	26 (76%)	551	177	172 (97%)
Nursing home physicians	50	44	43 (86%)	922	565	463 (82%)
Total	405	365	322 (80%)	7366	2220	2257 (102%)

1) Excluding one respondent whose interview was unusable

finding time to fill in the standard questionnaires. Eventually 80% of the initial respondents participated in the prospective study.

The average number of physician-weeks was less for the specialists working in hospitals than for the other respondents. This was due to the fact that specialists working in hospital were, on the whole, interviewed later in the study than general practitioners and nursing home physicians and therefore started with the prospective study at a later date. Together with the date of termination of the study on 31 May 1991 this led to a period of participation of less than 6 months for a greater number of respondents.

Completeness

The completeness of responses with respect to the number of deaths about which respondents supplied information is obviously important. The prospective study differed from the death certificate study in this respect. The death certificate study contained a sample of deaths, which permits the estimation of response percentages almost directly from the number of filled-in questionnaires. The response percentage of the prospective study could not be determined with certainty. However, the number of deaths occurring in a given group is known for the entire group of specialists of the particular specialty (Table C.1 and Table E.2). Based on this information one can estimate fairly accurately the proportion of deaths suitable for inclusion into the prospective study for which the respondent supplied information. That information is presented in Table C.7. The total number of deaths reported almost agrees with the expected number of deaths (2257 and 2220, respectively). The cardiologists reported a few more deaths than expected, the nursing home physicians somewhat fewer.

Representativity

Based on the information presented above it is likely that the data from the prospective study are reasonably complete. In the event that the data were incomplete it was very important to know if bias had occurred. For this purpose the study results were compared to the known data for the entire Netherlands. Table C.8 shows some characteristics of the deceased from the prospective study as compared to data for 1990 of The Netherlands.

The sex distribution of deaths is not quite identical to that for the entire Netherlands. There were relatively more deceased men in the prospective

Table C.8   Representativity of the prospective study (prospective study)

		Prospective study n=2257 %	The Nederlands, 1990[1]) n=128786 %
Sex	Males	54.0	51.7
	Females	46.0	48.3
	Total	100.0	100.0
Age	0 year	0.1	1.1
	1-19	0.9	0.8
	20-49	5.3	6.0
	50-64	13.5	13.1
	65-79	39.0	37.3
	80+	41.2	41.6
	Total	100.0	100.0
Cause of death	Cancer	26.1	27.3
	Cardiovascular diseases	35.4	30.4
	Diseases of the nervous system	11.9	11.7
	Pulmonary diseases	9.1	8.0
	External causes	2.4	4.1
	Mental disorders	1.4	0.9
	Others (all other categories)	13.7	17.6
	Total	100.0	100.0

1)   Source: CBS causes-of-death statistics.

study. The most obvious explanation can be found in the coding procedure used. The respondent had to select a code from a list in which sex and age were combined into one code. The design of the list of codes could have led some respondents to record wrongly the code for 'male' instead of for 'female'. There are, however, no important consequences for the distribution of the most important decisions. The age distribution agrees well with that for the entire Netherlands. This strengthens the expectation that no bias was introduced into the results of the prospective study.

The same can be said about the causes of death. There are numerous strict coding rules for the registration by the CBS of causes of death. The questions asked in the prospective study were not totally identical to those on the cause-of-death form although the formulations were identical for key issues. The slight differences in the distribution for causes of death can very easily be explained by the differences in coding procedures. One can conclude that there was no bias in the cause of death distribution. It is particularly important that cancer is not reported more often as cause of death in this study than for all deaths in The Netherlands. Considering the special position, according to this study, of this cause of death in MDELs this is an important indication that respondents have not filled in their questionnaires selectively for deaths for which MDEL-actions were performed.

The data from the physician interviews were used to search for a possible difference between the respondents who took part in the prospective study and those who eventually did not take part. There was no significant difference between the two groups as to the percentage of respondents indicating that they had at some point, or within the past 24 months, performed euthanasia or a life-terminating act without explicit request of the patient.

C.7 Comparison of the non-response in the three part-studies

The participation and refusal percentages presented above for the three part-studies are not fully comparable. In the death certificate study 24% of the questionnaires was not returned. The reasons for non-return are not known. It is probable that not only refusal of the respondent to participate, but long-lasting illness, change of work environment etc. may also have been involved. Taking into account stratum 0 this means that 27% of the sample data were in fact not observed.

To calculate a percentage for the physician interviews that can be compared to the above, one must not only consider the refusers, but also those with long-lasting illness, those in practice for less than two years as well as add a correction factor for the number of hospital deaths not covered by the five groups of specialists (Section E.2). The most comparable percentage for the physician interview then becomes 20%. This means that no information was in fact collected for about 20% of the domain about which we want to draw conclusions. This percentage is only partly due to refusal to participate. The greater part is a consequence, taken into account in advance, of the sampling procedure.

If one multiplies the participation rates for the three types of physicians in the prospective study with the percentages calculated as described above for the physician interviews, the comparable percentage for the prospective study becomes then 37%. This means that 37% of the intended sample data in fact were not observed.

The previous sections explored the possible sources of bias in the three part-studies. It was concluded that there are good reasons to assume that the observed distributions are also valid for the part of the sample that was not observed and that therefore the risk of bias is limited.

The interpretation of the questions of the standard questionnaire

Appendix D

D.1 Introduction

The framework of concepts used in the design of this investigation was discussed in Chapter 3. The design selected made it possible to follow the actual decisions and action of the physician, while also questions were asked as to the intention(s) behind the performance of certain actions. Concepts such as 'euthanasia' and 'assisted suicide' did not appear on the standard questionnaire. It was considered that the respondent probably has his own interpretation of these 'loaded' concepts, even if these concepts were described very carefully. The idea behind the formulations selected for the standard questionnaire was that one should be able to compare the various types of MDELs on the basis of the results: euthanasia, assisted suicide and acting to terminate life without explicit request had to be identified as distinct decisions and actions. This was discussed in more detail in Chapter 11 on the development of the standard questionnaire. It is also stated in this chapter that the answer to question 7 ("Was the death caused by the use of a drug prescribed, supplied or administered by you or a colleague with the explicit purpose of hastening the end of life or of enabling the patient to end his own life?") and the answers to subsequent questions could allow a distinction to be made between euthanasia, assisted suicide or acting to terminate life without explicit request, according to the interpretation described in Chapter 3.

It was very important to know how respondents interpreted the questions of the standard questionnaire, particularly questions 4 to 7. The interview study was used for this purpose. All respondents in the interview study were sent a copy of the standard questionnaire before the interview. They were asked to fill in the questionnaire for the most recent death they had experienced as treating physician, unless this death was a totally unexpected and sudden one. The filled-in standard questionnaire was discussed with the respondent at the beginning of the interview.

D.2 Implementation

In most cases the respondent had indeed filled in the standard questionnaire prior to the visit of the interviewer. The discussion of the standard

238

questionnaire was omitted in some cases in which the standard questionnaire had not been filled in in advance, and in situations in which only a very limited amount of time was available for the interview. The interviewers discussed a total of 370 standard questionnaires with respondents, with particular attention given to questions 4 to 7.

If at least one of questions 4 to 7 was answered in the affirmative, the interviewer had to decide whether this case had to be explored in greater depth at some time in the interview. This forced the interviewer to check whether an affirmative reply to, e.g., question 7 was interpreted by the respondent as euthanasia, assisted suicide or acting to terminate life without explicit request. The interviewer had to indicate if the respondent apparently had interpreted one or more of the questions 4 to 7 in such a manner that the answer to the particular question in fact better suited one of the other questions.

D.3 Results

No MDEL was taken in 104 of the 370 cases while, at the other extreme, 34 respondents replied in the affirmative to question 7. The total distribution of affirmative answers to the key questions of the standard questionnaire justifies the suspicion that in many instances respondents described a death in which an important decision was taken, instead of the latest (not acute) death. This distribution should therefore not be compared with those described in Chapters 13 and 15 about the results of the death certificate and prospective studies.

The results of this re-interpretation are summarised in Table D.1. This table should be understood as follows. It was determined for each death which was the last question of series 4 to 7 answered in the affirmative. This allows all deaths to be assigned to the last MDEL-action mentioned. Table D1 shows the last MDEL-actions involved. This procedure is a logical consequence of the structure of the standard questionnaire as discussed in Chapter 11: increasingly serious combinations of actions and intentions are referred to in questions 4 to 7.

In 29 of the 370 deaths the respondent supplied important new information with respect to the interpretation of the standard questionnaire. In all other cases there was a clear relation between the death described by the respondent and the filling in of the standard questionnaire. Most of these 29 cases involved a shift towards a less "serious" intention for the last-mentioned action.

239

Table D.1 Re-interpretation, after discussion between interviewer and respondent, of questions in the standard questionnaire

	Number	%	"subtract"	"add"	difference	%
No decision taken	104	28.1	4	1	-3	27.3
Taking into account the probability that the end of life is hastened by:						
4a. withholding a treatment	26	7.0	} 2	10	+8	13.0
4b. withdrawing a treatment	14	3.8				
4c. intensifying alleviation of pain and/or symptoms	82	22.2	1	2	+1	22.4
In part with the purpose of hastening the end of life by:						
5. intensifying alleviation of pain and/or symptoms	30	8.1	–	8	+8	10.3
With the explicit purpose of hastening the end of life by						
6a. withholding a treatment	34	9.2	} 12	7	-5	20.3
6b. withdrawing a treatment	46	12.4				
7. prescribing, supplying or administering a drug	34	9.2	10	1	-9	6.8
Total	370	100.0	29	29	0	100.0

It is particularly important that 9 of the 34 respondents who had replied in the affirmative to question 7, later made a comment related to this affirmative answer. In some cases the respondents felt that intensifying the alleviation of pain and/or symptoms with morphine was more appropriately classified as "in part with the purpose of hastening the end of life" than "with the explicit purpose". In some other cases the respondent indicated that, in spite of the affirmative reply to question 7, neither euthanasia, assisted suicide nor acting to terminate life without request were involved. An illustrative case description was given in Section 11.3. The interpretation of questions 6a and 6b is also described in Section 11.3.

Once these weighting factors have been applied the answers for the various specialties can be summed and estimates applicable to the entire Netherlands can be made for either the total group of seven specialties or for other combinations of these specialties.

Together, the five clinical specialties selected cover 88.8% of all hospital deaths. A correction for this factor also had to be made to arrive at estimates for the entire Netherlands. This was done by multiplying the weighted estimates for the clinical specialties by 1.127. This procedure implied the assumption that the remaining hospital deaths did not deviate significantly from the 88.8% with respect to MDELs. This is not unlikely, except for paediatric mortality that accounts for 2% of hospital deaths. This is discussed further in Chapter 16 and Section 13.8.

E.3 Numerators and denominators

Physicians were always asked in the sequence shown here if they had ever performed the MDEL concerned, when this had happened for the last time and, if this was more recently than 12 or 24 months ago, how often had they performed such an action during the past 12 months and the 12 months preceeding these. This was done in order to arrive at estimates for the entire Netherlands.

It was obviously important to avoid double counts. It often happens mainly in large clinical units, that several specialists are the treating physician for a particular patient simultaneously or in succession. In these cases MDELs will often be taken after consultations. A great overestimate would result if each physician counted as MDELs taken by himself all patients in whose treatment he was partly involved. The following measures were taken to avoid such overestimates.

All physicians were asked how many deaths in the twelve months preceding the interview, or for all of 1989, had been booked in their name. General practitioners were asked about the size of their practice in the past year and about the number of deaths that occurred in their practice and that had not occurred in hospital or nursing home. When the physician's "own" cases could not be separated from those of colleagues in a group practice, the question was asked as to how many physicians had shared the responsibility for these patients.

When asked about frequencies ("when for the last time?" and "how often during the past 12, or 24, months?") a respondent was always reminded emphatically to restrict the answer to decisions or deaths where he himself had been primarily responsible. In other words: the patient for whom the particular decision was taken or treatment performed, must also have been included in the number of deaths or admissions which were to be assigned to this respondent. In cases where no distinction from other treating physicians could be made and thus only a joint number of admissions or deaths could be reported these cases had to appear for the entire group of physicians. This implies that numerator and denominator had to refer exactly to the same group of patients. This procedure avoids most double counts. Nevertheless, it cannot be excluded that double counts did occur in a few instances. The number of MDELs may thus be slightly overestimated in the interview study.

E.4 Frequency estimates based on physician interviews

The occurrence of various types of MDELs in The Netherlands was estimated on the basis of two kinds of questions asked during the interviews. After the physician was asked if he ever had taken a certain type of decision and had given an answer in the affirmative, a question followed as to the last time he had taken such a decision. The physician was then asked how often in the past 12 months, and sometimes also, how often during the 12 months prior, he had taken such a decision. Based on the answers to these questions a frequency estimate with confidence interval and with application of the appropriate weighting factors considered can easily be derived for the entire Netherlands.

The question "when for the last time?" was also the basis for a frequency estimate. A special computer program was developed for this estimate as it required the use of rather complicated mathematical functions.

The estimates of the number of cases of euthanasia and other MDELs arrived at on the basis of these calculations agreed very well with the frequency estimates based on the 12- and 24-month question. This confirms the expectation that the data obtained through interviews led to reliable frequency estimates. For the sake of clarity only one series of frequency estimates is presented in this report. Because the data based on the "12- and 24-month" question were based on a larger number of events than the "when for the last time" question we assume that the estimates based on the former question will be somewhat more reliable. The second series of estimates is therefore not presented separately.

E.5 Weighting factors for the prospective study

A total of 80% of all respondents interviewed participated in the prospective study. Not all respondents were able to participate for the full six months. The calculation of the weighting factors in this case therefore differs from the previous calculations.

Here the calculation of the weighting factors has as point of departure "physician-weeks" rather than individual phyisicians. The number of weeks of participation was determined for each participating physician. The total number of physician-weeks for each specialty was then summed. Excluding holidays and periods of sickness, the total of physician-weeks for a given specialty in The Netherlands is the number of physicians in this specialty multiplied by 52. The weighting factor for the prospective study therefore was:

$$\frac{total\,number\,of\,physician\text{-}weeks\,in\,speciality}{number\,of\,physician\text{-}weeks\,for\,this\,specialty\,in\,the\,prospective\,study}$$

The information required for this calculation is presented in Table C.1. The weighting factors calculated are presented in column B of Table E.1. Application of the weighting factors of column B to the number of filled-in questionnaires returned in the prospective study provides an estimate of the distribution of deaths for the entire Netherlands as presented in column 3 of Table E.2.

By combining information from the causes-of-death registry of the CBS, data from the Dutch Information System on Hospital Care and day Nursing (LMR) and the Dutch Nursing Home Information System (SIVIS) one arrives at an estimate of the distribution of the total number of deaths in The Netherlands as shown in Table E.2, column 1.

Table E.2   Distribution of deaths in The Netherlands (see text for explanation)

	Assumed	Death certificate study-	Prospective study
General practitioners	53,400	52,900	58,100
Specialists	53,500	50,900	51,100
Nursing home phsycians	20,300	21,800	16,300
Others	1,600	3,100	–

This estimate was based on the results of the death certificate study and on information obtained from the interview study. This complicated procedure was required because the official CBS death certificate only mentions 'hospital' or 'elsewhere' as place of death. Deaths in nursing homes are often classified under 'elsewhere' but occasionally appear under 'hospital'. Moreover, no place of death is mentioned in more than 7% of of all death certificates. The LMR has a record of how many deaths occur for each specialty but a number of deaths recorded by the CBS as having occurred in hospital do not occur in LMR records. Such cases include, e.g., patients who had to be brought to hospital acutely and who died (e.g. because of accident or infarct) prior to administrative admission.

The number of deaths found for the three kinds of physicians in the death certificate study and the prospective study showed some differences (Table E.2, columns 2 and 3). Because the distribution of the several types of MDEL-actions was not the same for the various kinds of physicians (see Appendix F), the results from the two part-studies can not be compared directly. A second correction factor was therefore derived for the results of the prospective study. This factor equalises the distribution of the number of deaths per kind of physician in the prospective study with the distribution in the death certificate study thus allowing direct comparison between the studies. These weighting factors are listed in column C of Table E.1.

E.6 Weighting factors for the death certificate study

Both the original sample and the final response from the death certificate study were classified according to place of death, cause of death, sex and age in order to be able to correct for non-response, including a small number of questionnaires not sent out or unusable. This procedure yielded two four-dimensional tables (not presented). Each element was counted with the particular stratum weights. Stratum 0 was not counted. Based on the original sample weighted with the stratum weights for the various sample fractions, the table gives a first estimate for the population. The quotient of the weighted sample and the weighted response number yields a correction factor for the non-response for each combination of place of death, cause of death, sex and age. Here, the combinations with a weighted sample of less than 90 cases were first combined according to place of death and cause of death.

In the meanwhile the cause of death statistics gave exact information about the number of persons, listed according to age and sex, that had died during the reporting period.

If one combines the estimated numbers of stratum 0 with the estimated numbers of other strata and considers the non-response, there are small differences between these numbers and the numbers actually observed. This can be explained in part by the fact that a small number of cause-of-death certificates were not yet available when needed and in part because the estimated numbers are based on a sample and therefore subject to sampling fluctuations. A second correction factor was introduced to bring the numbers in the death certificate study in line with the numbers of the above mentioned tables. In those tables women aged 12 to 19 years were combined into one group with women aged 20 to 49 years.

The final factor used to extrapolate the response to the population is equal to the product of the weight of the stratum and the two correction factors. Technically, the application of these extrapolation factors amounts to the method of generalised poststratification. Only the second correction factor is of importance for stratum 0 units. The correction factors were determined individually for the returned questionnaires related to the deaths from the month of July and from the months of August to November.

E.7 Confidence intervals

A stratified sample was used in each of the three part-studies. This had to be taken into account when confidence intervals were calculated. It implies that weighting factors had to be calculated for all individual strata. In all studies these weighting factors led to a considerable increase of the numbers found in the sample. For each of the part-studies confidence intervals are computed for the estimated numbers and percentages, taking into account the consequences of stratification.

These confidence intervals are presented only occasionally in this report. The most important presentation is to be found in Table 17.1.

The fact that the address file of specialists contained a large number of addresses of physicians who did not meet selection criteria was not taken into account in the calculation of confidence intervals for the physician interviews and the prospective study. Therefore it is likely that the true confidence intervals for the physician interview and prospective studies are slightly greater than those shown in Table 17.1.

E.8 Characteristics of "most recent cases"

In the physician interviews several questions were asked about the most recent case for which the physician had taken a particular type of decision. In the tables concerning the physician interviews the distribution of the replies to these questions was considered as valid for all decisions of this type in The Netherlands. This implies that the collection of "last cases" is considered as an random sample of all cases of this type. This probably is not entirely correct. A physician who often takes a certain type of decision probably deals with a kind of case that differs from that treated by physician who very rarely takes that decision. Either case gets the same weight when this approach is followed. This turned out not to introduce any important bias when the characteristics of physicians with many cases of a certain type were compared with the characteristics of physicians with few cases of this type.

Comparison of the death certificate study and the prospective study

Appendix F

This appendix belongs to the text of Chapter 15. In that chapter the results of the prospective study are discussed and compared to the results of the death certificate study (Chapter 13). In order to facilitate understanding of the report the authors decided to present all comparative tables in the present appendix. It was considered that there is a high degree of similarity between the results of the two part-studies.

The tables derived from the prospective study will be presented first in all instances followed by the corresponding table from the death certificate study.

Table F.1 **MDEL-actions performed by the physician; comparison of prospective study with death certificate study**

	Prospective study		Death certificate study	
	Replies given total n¹)= 2257 %³)	of which as last mentioned MDEL-action n¹)= 2257 %	Replies given MDEL-action n¹)= 5197 %³)	of which as last mentioned MDEL-action n¹)= 5197 %
No MDEL-action performed	**64.6**	**64.6**	**60.6**	**60.6**
Stratum 0²)	n.a.	n.a.	9.0	9.0
First contact after the death	2.1	2.1	2.8	2.8
Sudden and totally unexpected death	29.2	29.2	18.1	18.1
Other cases where no MDEL-action was performed				
(no 'yes' to questions 4 to 7)	33.3	33.3	30.6	30.6
MDEL-action performed	**35.4**	**35.4**	**39.4**	**39.4**
Taking into account the probability that the end of life was hastened by:				
4a. withholding a treatment	19.6	5.5	21.6	5.6
4b. withdrawing a treatment	13.2	3.5	13.9	3.6
4c. intensifying alleviation of pain and/or symptoms	20.2	11.2	25.0	15.0
In part with the purpose of hastening the end of life by:				
5. intensifying alleviation of pain and/or symptoms	7.0	2.6	7.6	3.8
With the explicit purpose of hastening the end of life by:				
6a. withholding a treatment	7.2	3.5	7.1	4.3
6b. withdrawing a treatment	5.7	4.4	5.1	4.3
7. prescribing, supplying or administering a drug	4.7	4.7	2.7	2.7
Total	**100.0**	**100.0**	**100.0**	**100.0**

1. Total number of standard questionnaires on which this column is based (plus stratum 0 for the death certificate study).
2. Because no standard questionnaires had been sent of stratum 0 (death certificate study), the distribution over the next three categories is not known. It is known, however, that no MDEL-action was performed in these cases (see section 12.2 and the text of the standard questionnaire). In the death certificate study those 3 categories do not contain stratum 0 deaths.
3. The percentages in this column add up to more than 100%, because more than one of questions 4 to 7 could be answered with "yes".

Table F.2   Extent of shortening of life, based on last mentioned MDEL-action (prospective study)

	Last-mentioned MDEL-action[1])							
	4a n= 128 %	4b n= 77 %	4c n= 266 %	5 n= 55 %	6a n= 86 %	6b n= 101 %	7 n= 105 %	Total n= 818 %
Unknown	8	5	13	6	4	4	–	7
no shortening	35	33	42	19	9	13	2	26
<24 hours	3	18	19	32	7	24	24	17
I day to I week	26	27	19	25	33	26	28	25
I to 4 weeks	15	14	5	10	24	26	37	17
I to 6 months	10	2	2	7	24	7	7	7
>1/2 year	3	2	–	–	–	–	2	1
Total	100	100	100	100	100	100	100	100

Table 13.2   Extent of shortening of life, based on last mentioned MDEL-action (death certificate study)

	Last-mentioned MDEL-action[1])							
	4a n= 309 %	4b n= 204 %	4c n= 922 %	5 n= 244 %	6a n= 244 %	6b n= 234 %	7 n= 204 %	Total n= 2361 %
Unknown	13	17	17	2	5	3	I	11
no shortening	46	48	48	12	16	12	I	34
<24 hours	5	11	16	35	7	20	24	16
I day to I week	17	13	14	41	35	46	41	25
I to 4 weeks	11	8	4	9	24	14	19	10
I to 6 months	7	2	2	I	10	3	11	4
>1/2 year	I	0	0	–	3	1	3	1
Total	100	100	100	100	100	100	100	100

1)   Taking into account the probability that the end of life was hastened by:
    4a   withholding a treatment
    4b   withdrawing a treatment
    4c   intensifying alleviation of pain and/or symptoms
In part with the purpose of hastening the end of life by:
    5   intensifying alleviation of pain and/or symptoms
With the explicit purpose of hastening the end of life by:
    6a   withholding a treatment
    6b   withdrawing a treatment
    7   prescribing, supplying or administering a drug

Table F.3 Discussion with the patient about the decision to be taken, according to "last-mentioned" MDEL-action (prospective study)

	Last-mentioned MDEL-action[1])							Total with MDEL-action
	4a	4b	4c	5	6a	6b	7	
	n= 128	n= 77	n= 266	n= 55	n= 86	n= 101	n= 105	n= 818
	%	%	%	%	%	%	%	%
Discussed	26	34	29	44	34	47	78	40
Not discussed	69	61	58	50	64	49	22	54
Unknown	6	5	13	6	2	4	–	7
Total	100	100	100	100	100	100	100	100

Table 13.3 Discussion with the patient about the decision to be taken, according to "last-mentioned" MDEL-action (death certificate study)

	Last-mentioned MDEL-action[1])							Total with MDEL-action
	4a	4b	4c	5	6a	6b	7	
	n= 309	n= 204	n= 922	n= 244	n= 244	n= 234	n= 204	n= 2361
	%	%	%	%	%	%	%	%
Discussed	27	19	30	53	33	39	83	36
Not discussed	63	67	52	45	64	59	17	54
Unknown	9	14	18	2	3	2	–	10
Total	100	100	100	100	100	100	100	100

1) Taking into account the probability that the end of life was hastened by:

    4a withholding a treatment

    4b withdrawing a treatment

    4c intensifying alleviation of pain and/or symptoms

In part with the purpose of hastening the end of life by:

    5   intensifying alleviation of pain and/or symptoms

With the explicit purpose of hastening the end of life by:

    6a withholding a treatment

    6b withdrawing a treatment

    7   prescribing, supplying or administering a drug

Table F.4   Decision-taking after discussion with the patient, according to last-mentioned MDEL-action[1])(prospective study)

	Last-mentioned MDEL-action[2])					
	4a/b n=54 %	4c n= 83 %	5 n=25 %	6a/6b n= 70 %	7 n=78 %	Total n= 310 %
Decision taken upon explicit						
request by patient	47	48	64	68	85	64
Explicit and repeated request	37	38	60	51	83	54
Written advance directive	3	4	10	11	58	20
Patient totally able to take a decision	82	89	96	88	97	90
Initiative for discussion came from[3]):						
– patient	38	42	54	54	83	55
– physician (and not from patient)	58	56	22	43	16	40
In addition to discussion with patient there was discussion with[3])						
– colleagues	67	53	70	65	88	69
– nursing staff	51	63	72	50	49	55
– relatives	70	75	96	80	81	79
– no one	5	4	–	7	2	4

Table 13.4   Decision-taking after discussion with the patient, according to last-mentioned MDEL-action[1])(death certificate study)

	Last-mentioned MDEL-action[2])					
	4a/b n=136 %	4c n= 291 %	5 n=134 %	6a/6b n= 185 %	7 n=179 %	Total n= 925 %
Decision taken upon explicit						
request by patient	52	48	53	63	84	59
Explicit and repeated request	47	38	49	55	79	51
Written advance directive	3	3	10	6	42	11
Patient totally able to take a decision	83	84	84	75	96	84
Initiative for discussion came from[3]):						
– patient	41	39	58	46	74	49
– physician (and not from patient)	54	56	32	49	21	54
In addition to discussion with patient there was discussion with[3])						
– colleagues	57	58	60	62	81	63
– nursing staff	47	49	59	64	40	52
– relatives	65	70	77	82	87	76
– no one	9	8	5	2	2	6

1) Percentages in this table always refer to the total number of patients per last-mentioned action with whom this action had been discussed.

2) see 1) table F.2.

3) More than one answer could be given to this question.

Table F.5 Decision-taking without discussing with the patient, according to last-mentioned MDEL-action[1]) (prospective study)

	Last-mentioned MDEL-action[2])					Total
	4a/b n= 142 %	4c n= 157 %	5 n=27 %	6a/b n= 112 %	7 n= 27 %	n=465 %
No discussion possible	86	77	78	93	90	84
Patient unable to take a decision	80	70	78	91	88	80
Patient had at some time indicated a wish to hasten the end of life	2	9	35	13	33	11
An explicit request to hasten the end of life of patient by:						
− relatives	8	5	34	26	44	15
− physician/nurse/others (but not relatives)	1	−	−	1	3	1
− no one	91	92	61	73	53	83
Decision discussed with[3]):						
− colleagues	43	29	38	61	64	43
− nursing staff	61	54	56	77	57	62
− relatives	53	49	75	77	64	59
− no one	16	28	17	5	7	17

Table 13.5 Decision-taking without discussing with the patient, according to last-mentioned MDEL-action[1]) (death certificate study)

	Last-mentioned MDEL-action[2])					Total
	4a/b n= 321 %	4c n= 468 %	5 n=105 %	6a/b n= 282 %	7 n= 25 %	n=1201 %
No discussion possible	91	77	88	94	100	86
Patient unable to take a decision	87	72	77	88	85	81
Patient had at some time indicated a wish to hasten the end of life	11	9	22	16	25	13
An explicit request to hasten the end of life of patient by:						
− relatives	7	8	25	26	49	14
− physician/nurse/others (but not relatives)	0	1	1	2	3	1
− no one	84	84	70	67	49	78
Decision discussed with[3]):						
− colleagues	42	31	43	53	70	42
− nursing staff	55	36	58	66	79	51
− relatives	68	52	70	81	87	66
− no one	16	29	15	5	3	18

1) The percentages in this table always refer to the total number of patients per last-mentioned action with whom the action had not been discussed.

2) See 1) table F2

3) More than one answer coud be given to this question.

Table F.6 **Reasons for not discussing with the patient, according to last-mentioned MDEL-action[1]) (prospective study)**

	Last-mentioned MDEL-action[2])					
	4a/b n= 142 %	4c n= 157 %	5 n=27 %	6a/b n= 112 %	7 n= 27 %	Total n=465 %
Too young	1	1	–	–	–	1
Emotionally too labile (b)	3	5	4	1	7	3
Clearly the best for the patient (c)	13	25	24	15	25	19
Would have done more harm than good (d)	7	14	9	6	2	9
Only b and/or c and/or d and no other answering category (ability to take a decision not known)	13	18	14	7	7	13
Temporarily unconscious	3	2	9	2	–	3
Permanently unconscious	20	10	21	30	33	20
Reduced consciousness	33	41	38	43	50	39
Demented	38	29	24	28	19	31
Mentally handicapped	1	1	–	–	–	1
Mental disorder	5	5	11	1	2	4
Other reason	10	11	6	7	3	9
Unknown	–	2	5	–	–	1

Table 13.6 **Reasons for not discussing with the patient, according to last-mentioned MDEL-action[1]) (death certificate study)**

	Last-mentioned MDEL-action[2])					
	4a/b n= 321 %	4c n= 468 %	5 n=105 %	6a/b n= 282 %	7 n= 25 %	Total n=1201 %
Too young	2	1	1	4	9	2
Emotionally too labile (b)	1	2	5	1	3	2
Clearly the best for the patient (c)	11	28	27	14	26	20
Would have done more harm than good (d)	6	6	11	6	0	6
Only b and/or c and/or d and no other answering category (ability to take a decision not known)	7	17	18	6	8	11
Temporarily unconscious	4	3	1	5	–	4
Permanently unconscious	27	12	11	24	23	19
Reduced consciousness	39	46	57	42	57	44
Demented	32	22	23	32	11	27
Mentally handicapped	1	2	1	1	–	1
Mental disorder	5	2	–	2	3	2
Other reason	2	3	2	3	5	3
Unknown	4	6	4	2	8	4

1) More than one answer could be given to this question
2) See 1) table F2

Table F.7   Age and sex, according to last-mentioned MDEL-action (prospective study)

	MDEL-action	No MDEL-action	Last-mentioned MDEL-action[1])					All MDEL-actions together	Mortality in The Netherlands 1990[3])
			4a/b n= 205	4c n= 266	5 n= 55	6a/b n= 187	7 n= 105	n= 818	n=128786
	%[2])	%[2])	%	%	%	%	%	%	%
% last-mentioned action	35	65	9	11	3	8	5	36	
Age									
0-49	34	67	4	8	2	6	8	6	8
50-64	34	66	8	12	17	12	25	13	13
65-79	36	65	33	42	55	32	48	39	37
80+	59	41	55	39	26	50	20	42	42
Total	36	65	100	100	100	100	100	100	100
Sex									
Males	32	68	45	47	48	51	57	49	52
Females	40	60	56	53	52	49	43	51	48
Total	35	65	100	100	100	100	100	100	100

Table 13.7   Age and sex, according to last-mentioned MDEL-action (death certificate study)

	MDEL-action	No MDEL-action	Last-mentioned MDEL-action[1])					All MDEL-actions together	Mortality in The Netherlands 1990[3])
			4a/b n= 513	4c n= 922	5 n= 244	6a/b n= 478	7 n= 204	n= 2361	n=128786
	%[2])	%[2])	%	%	%	%	%	%	%
% last-mentioned action	39	61	9	15	4	9	3	39	
Age									
0-49	32	68	5	6	6	9	14	7	8
50-64	40	60	9	16	21	9	24	14	13
65-79	38	62	31	40	41	32	38	36	37
80+	42	58	56	38	32	50	25	43	42
Total	39	61	100	100	100	100	100	100	100
Sex									
Males	36	64	46	48	48	45	61	48	52
Females	43	57	54	52	52	55	39	52	48
Total	39	61	100	100	100	100	100	100	100

1)   See 1) table F2

2)   Row percentages

3)   Source: CBS causes-of-death statistics

Table F.8   Cause of death, according to last-mentioned MDEL-action (prospective study)

	MDEL-action	No MDEL-action	Last-mentioned MDEL-action [1]					All MDEL-actions together	Mortality in The Netherlands 1990[3]
			4a/b n= 205	4c n= 266	5 n= 55	6a/b n= 187	7 n= 105	n= 818	n=128786
	%[2]	%[2]	%	%	%	%	%	%	%
% last-mentioned action	35	65	9	11	3	8	5	36	
Cause of death									
Cancer	57	43	23	51	71	30	63	42	27
Cardiovascular diseases	17	83	23	16	14	19	5	17	30
Diseases of the nervous system (incl. stroke)	41	59	18	11	8	16	12	14	12
Pulmonary diseases	41	59	13	8	5	11	14	11	8
External causes	9	91	0.6	0.2	–	1.3	0.8	0.6	4.1
Mental disorders	52	48	2.6	1.7	–	3.7	–	2.0	0.9
Other (all other categories)	37	63	21	12	3	19	5	14	18
Total	36	65	100	100	100	100	100	100	100

Table 13.8   Cause of death, according to last-mentioned MDEL-action (death certificate study)

	MDEL-action	No MDEL-action	Last-mentioned MDEL-action[1]					All MDEL-actions together	Mortality in The Netherlands 1990[3]
			4a/b n= 513	4c n= 922	5 n= 244	6a/b n= 478	7 n= 204	n= 2361	n=128786
	%[2]	%[2]	%	%	%	%	%	%	%
% last-mentioned action	39	61	9	15	4	9	3	39	
Cause of death									
Cancer	59	41	28	53	61	31	68	44	27
Cardiovascular diseases	21	79	17	16	9	21	9	16	30
Diseases of the nervous system (incl. stroke)	43	57	21	9	10	15	2	13	12
Pulmonary diseases	37	63	9	5	8	8	6	7	8
External causes	12	88	1.5	1.1	1.8	1.2	0.3	1.2	4.1
Mental disorders	52	48	2.1	0.7	0.6	1.7	–	1.2	0.9
Other (all other categories)	43	58	21	16	9	23	15	18	18
Total	39	61	100	100	100	100	100	100	100

1) See 1) table F.2

2) Row percentages

3) Source: CBS causes-of-death statistics

Table F.9   Type of physician, according to last-mentioned MDEL-action[1]) (prospective study)

	Number of questionnaires processed	Last-mentioned MDEL-action[2])					MDEL-action	No MDEL-action	Total
		4a/b	4c	5	6a/b	7			
		%	%	%	%	%	%	%	%
% last-mentioned action		9.0	11.2	2.6	7.9	4.7	35.4	64.6	100.0
Type of physician									
General practitioner	618	7.1	9.9	2.8	5.8	6.8	32.4	67.6	100.0
Specialist	1176	8.5	8.8	2.7	9.3	4.3	33.6	66.4	100.0
Nursing home physician	463	15.1	19.9	2.2	9.7	0.4	47.3	52.7	100.0

Table 13.9   Type of physician, according to last-mentioned MDEL-action[1]) (death certificate study)

	Number of questionnaires processed	Last-mentioned MDEL-action[2])					MDEL-action	No MDEL-action	Total
		4a/b	4c	5	6a/b	7			
		%	%	%	%	%	%	%	%
% last-mentioned action		9.2	15.0	3.8	8.6	2.7	39.4	60.6	100.0
Type of physician									
General practitioner	2356	6.9	13.4	4.2	5.7	3.7	33.9	66.1	100.0
Specialist	1766	8.7	15.1	3.8	10.0	2.8	40.4	59.6	100.0
Nursing home physician	986	17.3	20.8	3.5	13.9	0.4	55.9	44.1	100.0
other (= other function and unknown)	89	1.7	1.0	–	0.5	0.6	3.8	96.2	100.0

1) In contrast to Tables 13.7 (F.7) and 13.8 (F.8), Table 13.9 (F.9) only has row percentages.

2) Taking into account the probability that the end of life was hastened by:
    4a withholding a treatment
    4b withdrawing a treatment
    4c intensifying alleviation of pain and/or symptoms
In part with the purpose of hastening the end of life by:
    5   intensifying alleviation of pain and/or symptoms
With the explicit purpose of hastening the end of life by:
    6a withholding a treatment
    6b withdrawing a treatment
    7   prescribing, supplying or administering a drug

Table F.10 Administration of a drug with the explicit purpose of hastening the end of life (prospective study)

	number n=105	weighted number n=5862	% of total n=125574
Administration (at least also) by physician	65	3940	3.1
Administration (also) by nurse (not by physician)	29	1112	0.9
Administration by others, not (also) by physician or nurse	3	193	0.2
Administration by patient, not (also) by physician, nurse or other	7	560	0.4
Unknown	1	57	0.05
Number of possible cases of euthanasia (see text)	53	3307	2.6

Table 13.10 Administration of a drug with the explicit purpose of hastening the end of life (death certificate study)

	number n=204	weighted number n=1125	% of total n=41587
Administration (at least also) by physician	151	775	1.9
Administration (also) by nurse (not by physician)	23	193	0.5
Administration by others, not (also) by physician or nurse	9	58	0.1
Administration by patient, not (also) by physician, nurse or other	17	82	0.2
Unknown	4	17	0.04
Number of possible cases of euthanasia (see text)	138	701	1.7

Table F.11   DNR decisions (prospective study)

	General practitioner n= 618 %	Specialist n= 1176 %	Nursing home physician n= 463 %	Total n= 2257 %
Explicitly agreed not to resuscitate[1])	15	61	18	34
− with colleagues	4	53	12	26
− with nursing staff	4	58	14	28
− with patient	7	8	3	7
− with relatives of patient	12	31	10	20
Only implicitly agreed	2	0	52	10
No DNR decision	81	37	31	54
Unknown	2	1	0	1
Total	100	100	100	100

1)   The agreement may have been made with one or more of the persons mentioned below.

Table 13.12   DNR decisions (death certificate study)

	General practitioner n= 2356 %	Specialist n= 1766 %	Nursing home physician n= 986 %	Total n= 5197 %
Explicitly agreed not to resuscitate[1])	16	60	28	35
− with colleagues	6	48	20	25
− with nursing staff	6	53	23	27
− with patient	8	9	6	8
− with relatives of patient	11	32	18	20
Only implicitly agreed	1	0	36	7
No DNR decision	80	38	33	56
Unknown	3	2	3	2
Total	100	100	100	100

1) The agreement may have been made with one or more of the persons mentioned below.

Table F.12 Requests to terminate life that were not carried out (prospective study)

	n= 2257 %
Explicit request that was not carried out [1]):	3.3
— yes, request by patient	2.5
— yes, request by relatives	1.0
— yes, request by others	0.1
No request that was not carried out	93.9
Unknown	2.8
Total	100.0

Table 13.13 Requests to terminate life that were not carried out (death certificate study)

	n= 5197 %
Explicit request that was not carried out [1]):	2.2
— yes, request by patient	1.4
— yes, request by relatives	1.1
— yes, request by others	0.1
No request that was not carried out	92.5
Unknown	5.3
Total	100.0

1) Request could have been made by one or more persons.